DR. CHRISTOPHER SEGLER
15-TIME IRONMAN FINISHER

RUNNING INJURY ROADMAP

The step by step guide any injured runner can use to resume workouts now and get back to running faster.

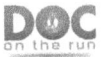

RUNNING INJURY ROADMAP

The step by step guide any injured runner can use to resume workouts now and get back to running faster

Copyright © 2020, Doc The Run, Dr. Christopher Segler, DPM - All Rights Reserved. No part of this work may be modified or altered in any form whatsoever, electronic, or mechanical, including photocopying, recording, or by any informational storage or retrieval system without express written, dated and signed permission from the author.

ISBN: 978-0-9965226-9-4

DOC ON THE RUN® is a registered trademark of Dr. Christopher Segler.

DISCLAIMER AND/OR LEGAL NOTICES: The information presented herein represents the view of the author as of the date of publication. Because of the rate with which conditions change, the author reserves the right to alter and update his opinion based on the new conditions. This book is for educational, entertainment and informational purposes only. While every attempt has been made to verify the information provided in this report, neither the author nor his affiliates/partners assume any responsibility for errors, inaccuracies or omissions. Any slights of people or organizations are unintentional. If advice concerning health, medical, surgical, legal or related matters is needed, the services of a fully qualified licensed professional should be sought. This book is not intended for use as, nor substitute for, a source of medical advice, legal or accounting advice. The use of this material or any exercises herein does not establish any physician-patient relationship. This book does not, nor is it intended to, serve as a substitute for professional medical advice, nor a consultation with a physician or qualified medical professional. You should be aware of any laws which govern health care and medical practices in your country and state. Any reference to any person or business whether living or dead is purely coincidental.

AFFILIATE DISCLAIMER. The short, direct, non-legal version is this: Some of the links in this book may be affiliate links which means that I earn money if you choose to buy from that vendor at some point in the near future. I do not choose which products and services to promote based upon which pay me the most, I choose based upon my decision of which I would recommend to a dear friend. You will never pay more for an item by clicking through my affiliate link, and, in fact, may pay less since I negotiate special offers for my readers that are not available elsewhere.

Cover design by Taofeek Abdulqoyum Abiola
Published by Virchow Press.
Printed in the United States of America.

RUNNING INJURY ROADMAP

TABLE OF CONTENTS

Introduction	page 1
Step 1: Define Your Goal	page 2
Step 2: Define "Healed"	page 5
Step 3: What Worked Before, Will Help Now	page 8
Step 4: Pain & Progress Are Your Guides	page 16
Step 5: Daily Tracking For 30 Days	page 21
Appendix 1: Runner's Pain Journal	page 82
Appendix 2: The Next Step	page 88

RUNNING INJURY ROADMAP
INTRODUCTION

What is most important to you, right now? Why do you need this road map? What do you want to accomplish with your running life? How can you use everything you know about running and apply it recovering from overtraining, injury and temporary setback? And yes, this setback is temporary. I promise.

After 20 years thinking about running injuries, more than 10 years of lecturing at medical conferences teaching doctors newer and better ways to treat inured runners, I have seen every possible mistake from doctors and runners alike.

Now listen closely...**You already know how to heal faster than normal.**

You probably ought to read that again.

Right now you have in your hands a tool to help you take a good look at your behavior, review your own knowledge base and decide how you can make some simple changes and daily commitments to heal faster.

I wrote this because most of what I do with runners isn't magical.

Yes, I have helped injured elite runners win world championships, place in national competitions and achieve once-in-a-lifetime goals. But all of the runners who were injured when we met, when we got to work: <u>they did the work</u>. Not me.

When injured elite runners call me, all I really do is listen closely, figure out what the problem is, help identify the most important goal, and then help them understand how the same training process that turned them into a successful runner can also turn them into a healed and fully recovered runner.

Most of training isn't really complicated. Most of healing isn't really complicated.

If you want to succeed in accelerating your healing, you need to apply everything that works in your training. Just take all the stuff you know and apply it to healing.

This book will take you through some written exercises to show you how.

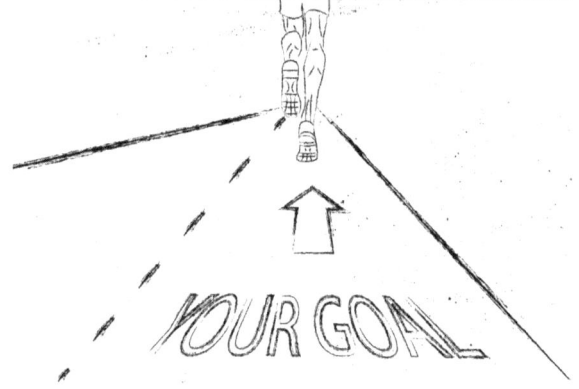

"PEOPLE WITH GOALS SUCCEED
BECAUSE THEY KNOW
WHERE THEY'RE GOING."

— EARL NIGHTINGALE

The very first step in healing is not figuring out your diagnosis or treatment. The first step is to pick your destination. You need a goal. You cannot plan a trip without a destination. And you cannot expect to heal as fast as possible if you do not have a clear goal and a defined timeline.

No doctor anywhere…not the one in your neighborhood…not the one who comes highly recommended by your running coach…not me…NO doctor can give you the best advice unless you have clarity on your running goals. If you don't have clarity on your running goals, do not expect any doctor to deliver the most effective treatment. Running injury treatment needs to be tailored to you, the severity of your specific injury and your running goals.

Goals are a compass. They provide you with direction on where you want to be, no matter where you start. Yes, even if you're injured, you need to start with a well-defined goal if you want faster-than-average progress.

You see, goals guide your daily actions because the end result you're working toward provides purpose for what you do on a daily basis.

Your already know this to be true. For example, if your goal was to run a marathon within 6 months, then the consistent actions of training daily and eating a healthy diet served a directed purpose toward that goal. Without that end goal in mind, we often lose motivation, feel aimless and lost. It's much harder to get out of bed to run, if you don't have a goal race in mind.

The same is true when recovering. You need to think about where you want to be. You need motivation to heal fast. Only then can you create a clear plan to get from where you are now, to where you want to go.

This book is designed to open your mind to the ways you can apply what you learned from running and recognize new opportunities for healing faster. You will develop and discover new paths to faster recovery.

But goals require commitment. **Commitment to the pursuit of rapid recovery is one of the greatest powers you have over any injury.**

As you flip through these pages, answer the written prompts honestly and thoughtfully. Doing so creates clarity about your injury and encourages you take action. Daily action is the fuel which accelerates your recovery.
Let's begin…

> *"If you fail to prepare, you're prepared to fail."*
> ~Mark Spitz, USA swimming gold medalist, 1972

STEP 1

PREPARE FOR THE JOURNEY

No one becomes a champion without believing success is achievable. The good news is that you are a runner. You already became a runner. You know you can do it. The bad news is right now, you probably feel down. You may even be wallowing in a little puddle of injury-induced self pity. Your confidence tank is running on empty. But you can fix that by just remembering and identifying with that healthy accomplished runner inside.

Prepare for your journey ahead, by looking back at past successes.

Think back to when you first decided to start running. When was it? Why did you decide to start running? Did you watch the Boston Marathon? Did you have a family friend who was an inspiring runner? What was it? Write down your original motivation and your reason for starting to run.

_____
_____

Think back to your first 5K or 10K or marathon, one that felt like your first "real run" that went well, when you first felt like you had put in the work, and completed and an event which defined you as a "real runner."

_____
_____

IF YOU HAVE TROUBLE WITH THIS, THEN JUST WRITE DOWN HOW YOUR NORMAL NON-RUNNER FRIENDS WOULD DESCRIBE YOU AS A RUNNER.
HOW WOULD YOUR FRIENDS DESCRIBE YOU, AS DIFFERENT FROM THEM?

_____
_____
_____
_____

Step 2
Define "Healed"

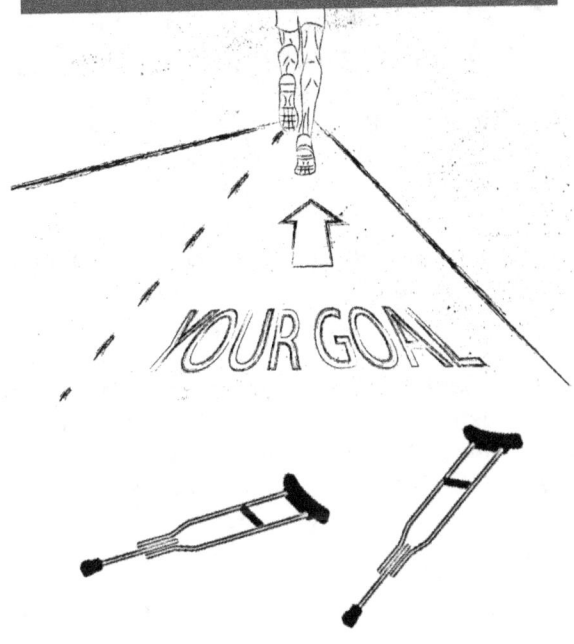

"THE QUESTION IS NOT HOW TO GET CURED, BUT HOW TO LIVE."

— JOSEPH CONRAD

"Our goals can only be reached through a vehicle of a plan, in which we must fervently believe, and upon which we must vigorously act. There is no other route to success."

— Pablo Picasso

STEP 2

DEFINE YOUR "GOAL RUN" THAT PROVES... "I'M HEALED!"

The very first thing I do when I talk to an injured runner who calls me for a web-cam virtual doctor visit or phone call coaching consultation is to try to clearly define that runner's "goal run." If you are injured, you probably aren't running. If you are running, you are probably not running as far, nor as fast as you really want. Instead, you're taking it easy, short and slow. In essence, you are dumbing-down your efforts just trying to not make things worse.

There is probably one particular long run, or maybe even a particular race that you cannot confidently do right now. But...if you could do that run, or finish that event, and enjoy it (instead of thinking about or worrying about your injury) you would be able to declare to yourself "I'm finally healed!"

Take a minute and think about your favorite weekly run or a dream race.

IF YOU DIDN'T HAVE ANY PAIN, WHAT WOULD BE YOUR "GOAL RUN"?
HINT: YOUR GOAL IS *NOT* TO GET RID OF THE FOOT PAIN!

FOCUS ON WHAT YOU REALLY WANT, WHAT YOU WOULD DO, IF YOU HAD NO PAIN.

(HOW FAR DO YOU WANT TO RUN, WHAT PACE? ON ROAD? ON TRAILS?)

IS THERE A SPECIFIC RUN OR EVENT YOU WOULD RACE? WHAT IS IT?

HERE ARE A COUPLE OF EXAMPLES:

"I AM GOING TO RUN 3-5 MILES, 5 DAYS A WEEK."
"I AM GOING TO RUN 10 MILES, FROM STINSON BEACH TO MUIR WOODS AND BACK."
"I AM GONG TO RUN THE CHICAGO MARATHON IN 3 HOURS AND 40 MINUTES."

WRITE IT DOWN...

HOW WOULD IT MAKE YOU FEEL TO ACTUALLY DO YOUR GOAL RUN?

WRITE IT DOWN, IN THE PRESENT TENSE, INCLUDING AS MUCH DESCRIPTION, FEELING AND VIVID EMOTION AS POSSIBLE.

AN EXAMPLE MIGHT BE:

"I RUN TO MUIR WOODS STARTING AT 2 O'CLOCK IN THE AFTERNOON WHEN THE SUN IS SHINING AND WARM ON MY SHOULDERS. I FEEL THE COOL OCEAN BREEZE, I CAN SMELL THE PINE TREES AND SAGE. I CAN FEEL THE CHANGING SOFTNESS OF THE TRAIL UNDERNEATH ME. MY QUADS ARE POWERFUL AND STRONG AS I RUN UP THE HILLS AND THE GRAVITY PULLS ME ALONG AS I RUN TO BACK DOWN. I FEEL STRONG AND ALIVE MOVING ACROSS THE MOUNTAIN."

___

VISUAL EXERCISE:

PRINT OUT AN IMAGE THAT CLEARLY REPRESENTS YOUR GOAL RUN. PUT IT ON YOUR MIRROR OR REFRIGERATOR WHERE YOU WILL SEE IT.

MORNING INTENTION EXERCISE:

EVERY MORNING, READ YOUR GOAL RUN STATEMENT ALOUD.

EVENING INTENTION EXERCISE:

EVERY EVENING, READ YOUR GOAL RUN STATEMENT ALOUD.

Step 3
What Worked Will Help Now

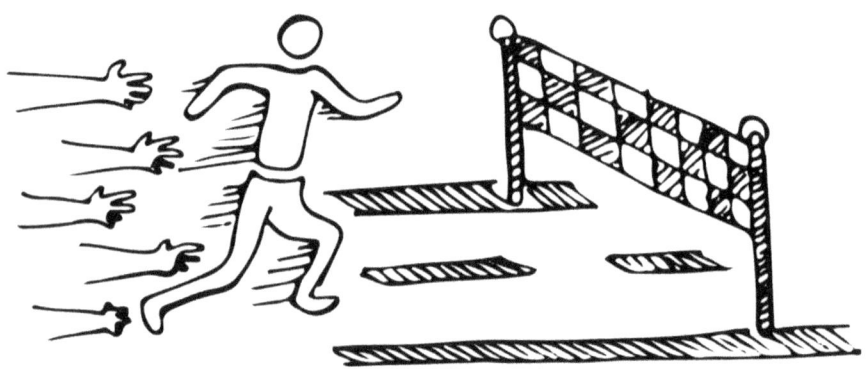

"WISDOM IS THE DAUGHTER OF EXPERIENCE."

— LEONARDO DA VINCI

Be very methodical in your life if you want to be a champion.
                                              -Alberto Juantorena

STEP 3

OUTLINE THE METHODS YOU USED TO TRAIN SUCCESSFULLY

Most injured runners who call me, they're back on their heels when injured. Deflated. Bummed. Scared. Cautious. Completely devoid of motivation and action. The "get up and go," has been replaced by "just sit here and wait."

The passive, "just wait for healing" approach is a soul killer for runners.

Runners who heal faster than expected do so because they apply themselves methodically in the same way they did when training for a race. You need to realize, remember...you know how to do the work of training.

It's time to shift your focus. Think about what you were doing to build your fitness right before you hit your last peak level of fitness. What did you do? Did you sit and hope for strength? Of course not...you worked your butt off!

But that work, called "training" is really just a simple process, applied daily.

You need to recognize and realize the process worked and it'll work again.

Think about what you did. You ran. You probably ran a lot. At some point you may have realized if you did a little core strengthening, that would help your running. Maybe you also added some strength training at the gym. Push-ups, planks, sit-ups. Yoga. Pilates. Swimming. What all did you add?

You spent time, attention, daily focus and you willed yourself to strength. Yes, it probably took a lot more than just long runs to get your running body in a state of maximum fitness and race-ready shape. But that's not all. You also probably did a lot of nutrition work, sleep focus and mental training. You trained every part of you that would support forward progress.

Take inventory of the efforts you put into your training and you will have a known, well-defined process you'll modify and apply to your recovery plan.

WHEN YOU WERE LAST RACE-FIT, AT YOUR MAXIMUM FITNESS, HOW MANY HOURS PER WEEK (AVERAGE) DID YOU SPEND DOING EXERCISE, TRAINING, & ACTUAL WORK OF GETTING STRONGER?
Write down all of the working out, types of sessions, and time in each. Add all the time on speed work, long runs, tempo runs, gym and cross-training. Take that total number of hours from a whole week of training and divide by 7 to get your daily average number of hours in training and exercising.

WHEN YOU WERE LAST RACE-FIT, AT YOUR MAXIMUM FITNESS, WHAT WAS YOUR NUTRITION PLAN AND DIET REGIMEN?
What did you eat. How often did you eat. Did you increase the frequency of meals or snacks to fuel the recovery from hard workouts? How many servings of fruits and vegetables, antioxidants and protein did you try to get in each day? What did you cut from your diet because it wasn't helping?

WHEN YOU WERE LAST RACE-FIT, AT YOUR MAXIMUM FITNESS, WHAT WAS YOUR SLEEP PLAN AND REGIMEN?
Did you have a goal, a plan or a tendency to get to bed earlier. Did you value and protect your sleep? Did you take naps? Did you have any habits like limiting screen time before bed when you were training and knew sleep really mattered?

___

WHEN YOU WERE LAST RACE-FIT, AT YOUR MAXIMUM FITNESS, WHAT WAS YOUR MENTAL FOCUS ROUTINE?
Did you visualize your goal being accomplished? Did you have any visual reminders of why you were putting in all of the hard work and dedication? Did you put your goal pace on your refrigerator? Did you set your marathon goal time as a screen saver on your phone? Did you create a vision board? Think of everything you did that helped your mental focus, visualization, inspiration that you thought might help motivate you to train.

___

Warning: This step of your self-analysis is going to be hard. It will feel raw. You must be honest to see how much or how little you have been doing (and are presently doing) to accelerate your recovery to get out of this rut.

IN THE LAST 3 DAYS, HOW MANY MINUTES PER DAY (AVERAGE) DID YOU SPEND DOING EXERCISE, ANYTHING YOU MAY CONSIDER "TRAINING," THE ACTUAL WORK OF GETTING STRONGER?
Write down all of the working out, types of sessions, and time in each. Add all time spent on yoga, core work, stretching, gym sessions, pilates, cycling, swimming, elliptical, any form of cross-training. Take that total number of hours from a whole week of training and divide by 7 to get your daily average number of hours in strengthening, training and exercising.
BE HONEST. IF THE ANSWER IS ZERO...WRITE IT DOWN.

_____
_____
_____
_____
_____

IN THE LAST 3 DAYS, WHAT DID YOUR DIET CONSIST OF?
What did you eat. Write down everything. Write down everything you ate that helped you heal faster. But also write down everything you put in your mouth that you know for a fact should be placed in the "cheating" column. Write down everything you ate, that you would eliminate from a running buddy's diet, if you were asked for advice on how you might make dietary improvements. How many servings of fruits and vegetables, antioxidants and protein did you get in each day? What should you cut from your diet because you know it is unhealthy and isn't really helping you heal? And yes...drinks count, too.
BE HONEST...WRITE IT ALL DOWN.

_____
_____
_____
_____
_____

IN THE LAST 3 DAYS, WHAT WAS YOUR SLEEP REGIMEN?
Did you a have a sleep quality goal, a plan or a tendency to get to bed earlier. Did you value and protect your sleep? Did you take naps? Did you have any habits like limiting screen time before bed?
BE HONEST. IF YOU WEREN'T DELIBERATE ABOUT SLEEP, OWN IT.

___

IN THE LAST 3 DAYS, WHAT WAS YOUR MENTAL FOCUS ROUTINE?
Did you visualize your goal being accomplished? Did you visualize your little fibroblast cells laying down collagen repairs, osteoblast cells repairing bone. Did you picture your blood flowing to deliver nourishing oxygen to your healing tissue? Did you picture your macrophage cells gobbling up damaged tissue to carry away the garbage that needs to be cleared out? Did you have any visual reminders of why you were putting in the work? Did you picture yourself healthy and running again? Did look at your next running goal? Think of everything you did that helped your mental focus, visualization, inspiration that you thought might help motivate you to heal.
BE HONEST. IF YOU JUST SAT AROUND BUMMED OUT, OWN IT!

NOW, LET'S SHIFT YOUR FOCUS BACK TO MORE POSITIVE ACTION.

LOOK AT YOUR TRAINING AND WORKOUTS BEFORE YOUR INJURY. THINK ABOUT EACH ONE YOU WROTE DOWN. WHICH ONES CAN YOU DO RIGHT NOW, WITHOUT MAKING YOUR INJURY WORSE?
WRITE ALL OF THEM DOWN HERE...

COME UP WITH 3 OTHER SPECIFIC EXERCISES THAT YOU COULD DO TO BUILD AEROBIC FITNESS, FLEXIBILITY, AND STRENGTH. COME UP WITH ONE IN EACH CATEGORY, ONES YOU CAN DO RIGHT NOW, WITHOUT MAKING YOUR INJURY WORSE.
WRITE ALL THREE OF THEM DOWN ADDING TO THE EXERCISES ABOVE.

TAKE INVENTORY OF YOUR DIET IN TRAINING, AND AFTER INJURY AND MAKE A LIST OF ALL THE WAYS YOU CAN IMPROVE IT NOW.
WRITE ALL OF THEM DOWN HERE...

COME UP WITH 3 MORE DIETARY ADDITIONS OR DELETIONS YOU WOULD EXPECT WILL HELP YOU HEAL FASTER THAT NORMAL.
WRITE ALL THREE OF THEM DOWN ADDING TO THE CHANGES ABOVE.

_____
_____
_____
_____
_____
_____
_____
_____

TAKE INVENTORY OF YOUR SLEEP PATTERNS, BEFORE AND AFTER INJURY. WHAT CAN YOU CHANGE TO GET BETTER SLEEP?
WRITE ALL OF THEM DOWN HERE...

_____
_____
_____
_____
_____
_____
_____
_____

TAKE INVENTORY OF YOUR MENTAL FOCUS ROUTINE BEFORE AND AFTER INJURY. WHAT ROUTINE CAN DO DAILY TO CLEARLY PICTURE YOUR CELLS REPAIRING AND VISUALIZE HEALING?
WRITE ALL OF THEM DOWN HERE...

_____
_____
_____
_____
_____
_____
_____
_____

Step 4
Pain & Progress are your guides

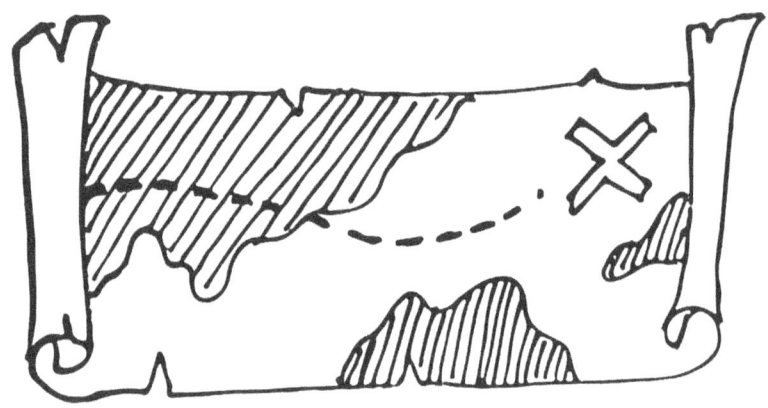

"ONCE YOU CAN LISTEN TO THOSE VOICES COMING FROM WITHIN, YOU ARE ACTUALLY GETTING CLOSER TO YOUR PASSION."

— DR. PREM JAGYASI

STEP 4

TRACK AND USE PAIN TO ADJUST COURSE IN RECOVERY

Pain is a tool to recover faster from running injury.

Today we are going to help you understand how a runner should measure pain so that you can us it as a tool in the injury recovery process. But you have to realize you and your perception of pain are not normal.

Runners are not normal.

Runner's pain levels are not normal.

Runners lack the sensitivity to pain that normal non-running patients feel.

These are all advantages when it comes to training and racing, but disadvantages when it comes to healing. But don't worry, there is a flip side to this equation that is a little more positive.

Runners have better somatic awareness than normal patients. You feel more nuances in the way your feet hit the ground and the way your legs feel when you are not having the best day. In a sense you feel musculoskeletal sensations better than average patients.

If you want to get back to running sooner, you need to advance your activity faster than the average patient. You also have to figure out a way to maintain the maximum level of activity your healing tissues can withstand without causing any further damage and without impeding the healing process.

If you are a runner and you want to heal an over-training injury that may normally takes 6 to 8 weeks to heal you have to think carefully. Do you really want to just sit around and let your fitness vanish while you wait for a month and a half to two months for that one injured part to heal?

It is possible to heal an injured structure without losing all of your fitness. But the only way that can happen is if you maintain the activity that supports and strengthens everything else. There is a fine line between healing while your running fitness diminishes and healing while simultaneously advancing your fitness.

You cannot evaluate this with an X-ray. You cannot evaluate it with an MRI or CT scan or any fancy test. However, If you understand the basics of how tissue heals you will quickly realize that there will be some response which clearly tells you whether or not you're doing too much activity.

Pain, bruising, and swelling are the most reliable indicators of too much tissue stress and tissue damage.

Bruising is the worst sign. If you do any activity and you get an increase in bruising that means you did so much tissue damage that you actually had bleeding underneath the skin. Clearly that indicates way too much stress on the injured tissue. You are doing damage.

Second on the list is swelling. Swelling is fluid from inflammation. If you do too much activity and the next day you have an increase in swelling in your foot, then you definitely did too much activity the day before. It's inflamed!

Both bruising and swelling are both signs you did too much. If you keep doing those things that caused the bruising and swelling, you will definitely increase the damage to the healing tissue and delay your recovery.

Pain is a much more sensitive indicator. When it comes to healing and trying to figure out the line between too much activity and not enough activity, pain is your guide.

Normally doctors tell patients to look for pain and rate it on a number scale of 1 to 10. A pain level of 1 is just minimal discomfort, almost unnoticeable. A pain level of 10 would be excruciating. Think of somebody chopping off your leg with a dull axe.

Interestingly, in the last 15 years I don't think I have seen a single runner with an injury who said they had a 10 out of 10 pain level. I even saw a woman who broke her tibia in half and only called it an 8/10 pain.

The reason you and most runners don't seem to note a high level of pain when injured is that you, as a runner have learned how to tune out pain and ignore it. You taught yourself pain tolerance.

You ignore pain when you do hill repeats. You ignore pain when you run stairs. You tune out the pain and focus when you do speed work. And you shut out the painful noise in your legs when you are finishing a marathon.

Through the magic of neuroplasticity you have habituated yourself to down code your pain. But you still have to try to look for, identify, rate your pain consistently and accurately if you want to stay active and keep healing.

You have to know where the line is. You have to be able to recognize the pain level which could cause damage. An increase in pain obviously signifies more stress and probable tissue damage to the healing injury.

But a decrease in pain, a decrease in tenderness, signifies healing and increased tissue stability that can justify a slight increase in your activity level. But you have to look for the small changes in those pain levels. As a runner who has learned to ignore high levels of pain, this job can be difficult. But it is absolutely necessary if you really want to advance your fitness ahead of schedule.

Your job in looking for pain and soreness is to put a number on it.

If you think your pain is a 3 out of 10, but the next day you notice you actually have swelling, you did way too much activity and you were causing enough tissue damage to get rebound inflammation and swelling. So my guess is that a normal patient would've called that level of discomfort something more like a seven, eight, or nine out of 10 pain.

Over and over runners tell me they don't really have pain, but they only feel some "discomfort." You can call it whatever you want, but you have to be able to assign a level of pain or a level of discomfort that you can track.

Just yesterday I was doing a phone consultation call with a runner who was trying to figure out whether or not she could transition off of her crutches. She tried walking around and putting 25% of her weight on the injured foot, while protected in a fracture walking boot. She said she had no pain. She said, "I would not really call it any pain at all, it was really just discomfort."

But she noticed the next day she actually had swelling in her foot when she woke up. So my guess is her description of "discomfort" would be definitely described as "pain" by a normal patient. Of course her question was, "Should I just keep going with crutches and 25% of my weight on the foot, since it was only discomfort."

My answer was, "No way! You felt like it was only 'discomfort' but you had swelling indicating it was enough trouble to stimulate an inflammatory response." You will not heal with the continuing inflammatory response. So you have to back off if you see swelling.

In a similar way, you have to back off if you feel pain. So if she feels like that 25% pressure causes a 2/10 pain level, then her job is to realize 2/10 on her pain scale is too much. She needs to start looking for a decrease to a 1.5/10 pain. Although it may seem tedious to look for the very small changes in pain level as you progress, I promise it is worth the effort.

You only have a couple of options when you are healing a running injury. One option is to wait the prescribed 6 to 8 weeks and let that metatarsal stress fracture, sprained ankle ligament or Achilles tendon completely heal. If you wait that long to heal you will completely decimate your running fitness. And it will take many months to earn your running fitness back.

Another option is to figure out how to start strengthening all of the non-injured structures sooner. The only way to do that is to move them and use them without causing further damage to the healing bone, tendon or ligament. You have to keep everything else healthy if you don't want to lose your fitness.

Properly tracked pain is your guide in that process.

As soon as your pain level decreases you have a clear indication that the tissue is healing. There's a little bit more collagen stabilizing the injury. If you have little bit more inherent strength, you can move just a little bit more without sustaining any damage. If you push it just a little bit too far and you can recognize the subtle difference in discomfort (or pain) then you know where the line is, and you know when to back off or decrease activity.

Pay attention. Keep track. Look for the subtleties and the changes in your pain level. Make note daily and you will get back to running sooner.

Step 5
Daily Tracking

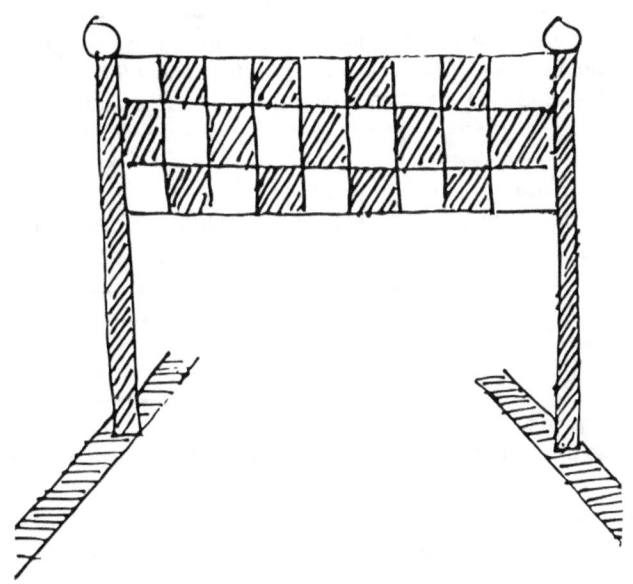

"WHAT YOU STAY FOCUSED ON WILL GROW."

— ROY T. BENNETT

Morning Recovery Preparation Exercises DAY 1 Date:_____

My goal run is:

Once I can do that run, I will know I am recovered!

Visualize cells in your body healing, repairing, making you stronger & rebuilding tissue. Close your eyes for 1 minute and visualize the healing now.

Visualize running your goal run. Picture the scene moving by, feel the air around you and think about how it will feel as you powerfully and effortlessly glide through the run. Close your eyes for 1 minute and visualize running now.

Daily Pain Assessment:
Notice and write down any pain, stiffness or discomfort you feel this morning.
_____
_____
_____
_____

Recognize progress:
How have these uncomfortable feelings diminished or improved over the past week?
_____
_____
_____

Nutrition Plan to Fuel Today's Recovery. What/when will you eat/drink today:

Breakfast:_____ a.m.
Morning snack or mini-meal: _____ a.m.
Lunch: _____ p.m.
Afternoon snack or mini-meal:_____ p.m.
Dinner:_____ p.m.
Fluids:_____
Most of my antioxidants will come from: _____
Injury recovery specific supplements: _____

Active Recovery Plan to Fuel Today's Progress.
What will I commit to doing today to strengthen and support my one injured part?
Legs:_____
Core: _____
Upper body: _____
NO-Load Aerobic exercises: _____
Low-Load Aerobic exercises: _____
Stretching:_____
Massage: _____
Other: _____

Evening Recognizing Recovery Exercises

Today I supported and protected my injury so it can keep healing.
What did I do to protect my injury during today's activities?
_____
_____

Today I prepared my whole body, making it stronger so it can better support my injury. What exercises did I do today that will me stronger and increase my fitness?
_____
_____

Today I fueled my body with healing nutrients.
What did I eat and drink today that will help my tissues heal and grow while I sleep tonight?
_____
_____

Prep your body to repair while you sleep
2 minute Nightly Visualization

Visualize running your goal run. Picture the scene moving by, feel the air around you and think about how it will feel as you powerfully and effortlessly glide through the run.
Before you go to sleep, close your eyes for 1 minute and visualize running now.

Visualize cells in your body healing, repairing, making you stronger & rebuilding tissue.
Before you go to sleep....
Close your eyes for 1 minute and visualize the healing now.

Morning Recovery Preparation Exercises DAY 2 Date:_____

My goal run is:

Once I can do that run, I will know I am recovered!

Visualize cells in your body healing, repairing, making you stronger & rebuilding tissue. Close your eyes for 1 minute and visualize the healing now.

Visualize running your goal run. Picture the scene moving by, feel the air around you and think about how it will feel as you powerfully and effortlessly glide through the run. Close your eyes for 1 minute and visualize running now.

Daily Pain Assessment:
Notice and write down any pain, stiffness or discomfort you feel this morning.
_____
_____
_____
_____

Recognize progress:
How have these uncomfortable feelings diminished or improved over the past week?
_____
_____
_____

Nutrition Plan to Fuel Today's Recovery. What/when will you eat/drink today:

Breakfast:_____ a.m.
Morning snack or mini-meal: _____ a.m.
Lunch: _____ p.m.
Afternoon snack or mini-meal:_____ p.m.
Dinner:_____ p.m.
Fluids:_____
Most of my antioxidants will come from: _____
Injury recovery specific supplements: _____

Active Recovery Plan to Fuel Today's Progress.
What will I commit to doing today to strengthen and support my one injured part?
Legs:_____
Core: _____
Upper body: _____
NO-Load Aerobic exercises: _____
Low-Load Aerobic exercises: _____
Stretching:_____
Massage: _____
Other: _____

Evening Recognizing Recovery Exercises

Today I supported and protected my injury so it can keep healing.
What did I do to protect my injury during today's activities?
_____
_____

Today I prepared my whole body, making it stronger so it can better support my injury. What exercises did I do today that will me stronger and increase my fitness?
_____
_____

Today I fueled my body with healing nutrients.
What did I eat and drink today that will help my tissues heal and grow while I sleep tonight?
_____
_____

Prep your body to repair while you sleep
2 minute Nightly Visualization

Visualize running your goal run. Picture the scene moving by, feel the air around you and think about how it will feel as you powerfully and effortlessly glide through the run.
Before you go to sleep, close your eyes for 1 minute and visualize running now.

Visualize cells in your body healing, repairing, making you stronger & rebuilding tissue.
Before you go to sleep....
Close your eyes for 1 minute and visualize the healing now.

Morning Recovery Preparation Exercises DAY 3 Date:_____

My goal run is:

Once I can do that run, I will know I am recovered!

Visualize cells in your body healing, repairing, making you stronger & rebuilding tissue. Close your eyes for 1 minute and visualize the healing now.

Visualize running your goal run. Picture the scene moving by, feel the air around you and think about how it will feel as you powerfully and effortlessly glide through the run. Close your eyes for 1 minute and visualize running now.

Daily Pain Assessment:
Notice and write down any pain, stiffness or discomfort you feel this morning.
_____
_____
_____
_____

Recognize progress:
How have these uncomfortable feelings diminished or improved over the past week?
_____
_____
_____

Nutrition Plan to Fuel Today's Recovery. What/when will you eat/drink today:

Breakfast:_____ a.m.
Morning snack or mini-meal: _____ a.m.
Lunch: _____ p.m.
Afternoon snack or mini-meal:_____ p.m.
Dinner:_____ p.m.
Fluids:_____
Most of my antioxidants will come from: _____
Injury recovery specific supplements: _____

Active Recovery Plan to Fuel Today's Progress.
What will I commit to doing today to strengthen and support my one injured part?
Legs:_____
Core: _____
Upper body: _____
NO-Load Aerobic exercises: _____
Low-Load Aerobic exercises: _____
Stretching:_____
Massage: _____
Other: _____

Evening Recognizing Recovery Exercises

Today I supported and protected my injury so it can keep healing.
What did I do to protect my injury during today's activities?
_____
_____

Today I prepared my whole body, making it stronger so it can better support my injury. What exercises did I do today that will me stronger and increase my fitness?
_____
_____

Today I fueled my body with healing nutrients.
What did I eat and drink today that will help my tissues heal and grow while I sleep tonight?
_____
_____

Prep your body to repair while you sleep
2 minute Nightly Visualization

Visualize running your goal run. Picture the scene moving by, feel the air around you and think about how it will feel as you powerfully and effortlessly glide through the run.
Before you go to sleep, close your eyes for 1 minute and visualize running now.

Visualize cells in your body healing, repairing, making you stronger & rebuilding tissue.
Before you go to sleep....
Close your eyes for 1 minute and visualize the healing now.

Morning Recovery Preparation Exercises DAY 4 Date:_____

My goal run is:

Once I can do that run, I will know I am recovered!

Visualize cells in your body healing, repairing, making you stronger & rebuilding tissue. Close your eyes for 1 minute and visualize the healing now.

Visualize running your goal run. Picture the scene moving by, feel the air around you and think about how it will feel as you powerfully and effortlessly glide through the run. Close your eyes for 1 minute and visualize running now.

Daily Pain Assessment:
Notice and write down any pain, stiffness or discomfort you feel this morning.
_____
_____
_____
_____

Recognize progress:
How have these uncomfortable feelings diminished or improved over the past week?
_____
_____
_____

Nutrition Plan to Fuel Today's Recovery. What/when will you eat/drink today:

Breakfast:_____ a.m.
Morning snack or mini-meal: _____ a.m.
Lunch: _____ p.m.
Afternoon snack or mini-meal:_____ p.m.
Dinner:_____ p.m.
Fluids:_____
Most of my antioxidants will come from: _____
Injury recovery specific supplements: _____

Active Recovery Plan to Fuel Today's Progress.
What will I commit to doing today to strengthen and support my one injured part?
Legs:_____
Core: _____
Upper body: _____
NO-Load Aerobic exercises: _____
Low-Load Aerobic exercises: _____
Stretching:_____
Massage: _____
Other: _____

Evening Recognizing Recovery Exercises

Today I supported and protected my injury so it can keep healing.
What did I do to protect my injury during today's activities?
_____
_____

Today I prepared my whole body, making it stronger so it can better support my injury. What exercises did I do today that will me stronger and increase my fitness?
_____
_____

Today I fueled my body with healing nutrients.
What did I eat and drink today that will help my tissues heal and grow while I sleep tonight?
_____
_____

Prep your body to repair while you sleep
2 minute Nightly Visualization

Visualize running your goal run. Picture the scene moving by, feel the air around you and think about how it will feel as you powerfully and effortlessly glide through the run. Before you go to sleep, close your eyes for 1 minute and visualize running now.

Visualize cells in your body healing, repairing, making you stronger & rebuilding tissue. Before you go to sleep....
Close your eyes for 1 minute and visualize the healing now.

Morning Recovery Preparation Exercises DAY 5 Date:_____

My goal run is:

Once I can do that run, I will know I am recovered!

Visualize cells in your body healing, repairing, making you stronger & rebuilding tissue. Close your eyes for 1 minute and visualize the healing now.

Visualize running your goal run. Picture the scene moving by, feel the air around you and think about how it will feel as you powerfully and effortlessly glide through the run. Close your eyes for 1 minute and visualize running now.

Daily Pain Assessment:
Notice and write down any pain, stiffness or discomfort you feel this morning.
_____
_____
_____
_____

Recognize progress:
How have these uncomfortable feelings diminished or improved over the past week?
_____
_____
_____

Nutrition Plan to Fuel Today's Recovery. What/when will you eat/drink today:

Breakfast:_____ a.m.
Morning snack or mini-meal: _____ a.m.
Lunch: _____ p.m.
Afternoon snack or mini-meal:_____ p.m.
Dinner:_____ p.m.
Fluids:_____
Most of my antioxidants will come from: _____
Injury recovery specific supplements: _____

Active Recovery Plan to Fuel Today's Progress.
What will I commit to doing today to strengthen and support my one injured part?
Legs:_____
Core: _____
Upper body: _____
NO-Load Aerobic exercises: _____
Low-Load Aerobic exercises: _____
Stretching:_____
Massage: _____
Other: _____

Evening Recognizing Recovery Exercises

Today I supported and protected my injury so it can keep healing.
What did I do to protect my injury during today's activities?
_____
_____

Today I prepared my whole body, making it stronger so it can better support my injury. What exercises did I do today that will me stronger and increase my fitness?
_____
_____

Today I fueled my body with healing nutrients.
What did I eat and drink today that will help my tissues heal and grow while I sleep tonight?
_____
_____

Prep your body to repair while you sleep
2 minute Nightly Visualization

Visualize running your goal run. Picture the scene moving by, feel the air around you and think about how it will feel as you powerfully and effortlessly glide through the run.
Before you go to sleep, close your eyes for 1 minute and visualize running now.

Visualize cells in your body healing, repairing, making you stronger & rebuilding tissue.
Before you go to sleep....
Close your eyes for 1 minute and visualize the healing now.

Morning Recovery Preparation Exercises DAY 6 Date:_____

My goal run is:

Once I can do that run, I will know I am recovered!

Visualize cells in your body healing, repairing, making you stronger & rebuilding tissue. Close your eyes for 1 minute and visualize the healing now.

Visualize running your goal run. Picture the scene moving by, feel the air around you and think about how it will feel as you powerfully and effortlessly glide through the run. Close your eyes for 1 minute and visualize running now.

Daily Pain Assessment:
Notice and write down any pain, stiffness or discomfort you feel this morning.
_____
_____
_____
_____

Recognize progress:
How have these uncomfortable feelings diminished or improved over the past week?
_____
_____
_____

Nutrition Plan to Fuel Today's Recovery. What/when will you eat/drink today:

Breakfast:_____ a.m.
Morning snack or mini-meal: _____ a.m.
Lunch: _____ p.m.
Afternoon snack or mini-meal:_____ p.m.
Dinner:_____ p.m.
Fluids:_____
Most of my antioxidants will come from: _____
Injury recovery specific supplements: _____

Active Recovery Plan to Fuel Today's Progress.
What will I commit to doing today to strengthen and support my one injured part?
Legs:_____
Core: _____
Upper body: _____
NO-Load Aerobic exercises: _____
Low-Load Aerobic exercises: _____
Stretching:_____
Massage: _____
Other: _____

Evening Recognizing Recovery Exercises

Today I supported and protected my injury so it can keep healing.
What did I do to protect my injury during today's activities?
_____
_____

Today I prepared my whole body, making it stronger so it can better support my injury. What exercises did I do today that will me stronger and increase my fitness?
_____
_____

Today I fueled my body with healing nutrients.
What did I eat and drink today that will help my tissues heal and grow while I sleep tonight?
_____
_____

Prep your body to repair while you sleep
2 minute Nightly Visualization

Visualize running your goal run. Picture the scene moving by, feel the air around you and think about how it will feel as you powerfully and effortlessly glide through the run.
Before you go to sleep, close your eyes for 1 minute and visualize running now.

Visualize cells in your body healing, repairing, making you stronger & rebuilding tissue.
Before you go to sleep….
Close your eyes for 1 minute and visualize the healing now.

Morning Recovery Preparation Exercises DAY 7 Date:_____

My goal run is:

Once I can do that run, I will know I am recovered!

Visualize cells in your body healing, repairing, making you stronger & rebuilding tissue. Close your eyes for 1 minute and visualize the healing now.

Visualize running your goal run. Picture the scene moving by, feel the air around you and think about how it will feel as you powerfully and effortlessly glide through the run. Close your eyes for 1 minute and visualize running now.

Daily Pain Assessment:
Notice and write down any pain, stiffness or discomfort you feel this morning.
_____
_____
_____
_____

Recognize progress:
How have these uncomfortable feelings diminished or improved over the past week?
_____
_____
_____

Nutrition Plan to Fuel Today's Recovery. What/when will you eat/drink today:

Breakfast:_____ a.m.
Morning snack or mini-meal: _____ a.m.
Lunch: _____ p.m.
Afternoon snack or mini-meal:_____ p.m.
Dinner:_____ p.m.
Fluids:_____
Most of my antioxidants will come from: _____
Injury recovery specific supplements: _____

Active Recovery Plan to Fuel Today's Progress.
What will I commit to doing today to strengthen and support my one injured part?
Legs:_____
Core: _____
Upper body: _____
NO-Load Aerobic exercises: _____
Low-Load Aerobic exercises: _____
Stretching:_____
Massage: _____
Other: _____

Evening Recognizing Recovery Exercises

Today I supported and protected my injury so it can keep healing.
What did I do to protect my injury during today's activities?
_____
_____

Today I prepared my whole body, making it stronger so it can better support my injury. What exercises did I do today that will me stronger and increase my fitness?
_____
_____

Today I fueled my body with healing nutrients.
What did I eat and drink today that will help my tissues heal and grow while I sleep tonight?
_____
_____

Prep your body to repair while you sleep
2 minute Nightly Visualization

Visualize running your goal run. Picture the scene moving by, feel the air around you and think about how it will feel as you powerfully and effortlessly glide through the run.
Before you go to sleep, close your eyes for 1 minute and visualize running now.

Visualize cells in your body healing, repairing, making you stronger & rebuilding tissue.
Before you go to sleep….
Close your eyes for 1 minute and visualize the healing now.

Morning Recovery Preparation Exercises DAY 8 Date:_____

My goal run is:

Once I can do that run, I will know I am recovered!

Visualize cells in your body healing, repairing, making you stronger & rebuilding tissue. Close your eyes for 1 minute and visualize the healing now.

Visualize running your goal run. Picture the scene moving by, feel the air around you and think about how it will feel as you powerfully and effortlessly glide through the run. Close your eyes for 1 minute and visualize running now.

Daily Pain Assessment:
Notice and write down any pain, stiffness or discomfort you feel this morning.
_____
_____
_____
_____

Recognize progress:
How have these uncomfortable feelings diminished or improved over the past week?
_____
_____
_____

Nutrition Plan to Fuel Today's Recovery. What/when will you eat/drink today:

Breakfast:_____ a.m.
Morning snack or mini-meal: _____ a.m.
Lunch: _____ p.m.
Afternoon snack or mini-meal:_____ p.m.
Dinner:_____ p.m.
Fluids:_____
Most of my antioxidants will come from: _____
Injury recovery specific supplements: _____

Active Recovery Plan to Fuel Today's Progress.
What will I commit to doing today to strengthen and support my one injured part?
Legs:_____
Core: _____
Upper body: _____
NO-Load Aerobic exercises: _____
Low-Load Aerobic exercises: _____
Stretching:_____
Massage: _____
Other: _____

Evening Recognizing Recovery Exercises

Today I supported and protected my injury so it can keep healing.
What did I do to protect my injury during today's activities?
_____
_____

Today I prepared my whole body, making it stronger so it can better support my injury. What exercises did I do today that will me stronger and increase my fitness?
_____
_____

Today I fueled my body with healing nutrients.
What did I eat and drink today that will help my tissues heal and grow while I sleep tonight?
_____
_____

Prep your body to repair while you sleep
2 minute Nightly Visualization

Visualize running your goal run. Picture the scene moving by, feel the air around you and think about how it will feel as you powerfully and effortlessly glide through the run.
Before you go to sleep, close your eyes for 1 minute and visualize running now.

Visualize cells in your body healing, repairing, making you stronger & rebuilding tissue.
Before you go to sleep....
Close your eyes for 1 minute and visualize the healing now.

Morning Recovery Preparation Exercises DAY 9 Date:_____

My goal run is:

Once I can do that run, I will know I am recovered!

Visualize cells in your body healing, repairing, making you stronger & rebuilding tissue. Close your eyes for 1 minute and visualize the healing now.

Visualize running your goal run. Picture the scene moving by, feel the air around you and think about how it will feel as you powerfully and effortlessly glide through the run. Close your eyes for 1 minute and visualize running now.

Daily Pain Assessment:
Notice and write down any pain, stiffness or discomfort you feel this morning.
_____
_____
_____
_____

Recognize progress:
How have these uncomfortable feelings diminished or improved over the past week?
_____
_____
_____
_____

Nutrition Plan to Fuel Today's Recovery. What/when will you eat/drink today:

Breakfast:_____ a.m.
Morning snack or mini-meal: _____ a.m.
Lunch: _____ p.m.
Afternoon snack or mini-meal:_____ p.m.
Dinner:_____ p.m.
Fluids:_____
Most of my antioxidants will come from: _____
Injury recovery specific supplements: _____

Active Recovery Plan to Fuel Today's Progress.
What will I commit to doing today to strengthen and support my one injured part?
Legs:_____
Core: _____
Upper body: _____
NO-Load Aerobic exercises: _____
Low-Load Aerobic exercises: _____
Stretching:_____
Massage: _____
Other: _____

Evening Recognizing Recovery Exercises

Today I supported and protected my injury so it can keep healing.
What did I do to protect my injury during today's activities?
_____
_____

Today I prepared my whole body, making it stronger so it can better support my injury. What exercises did I do today that will me stronger and increase my fitness?
_____
_____

Today I fueled my body with healing nutrients.
What did I eat and drink today that will help my tissues heal and grow while I sleep tonight?
_____
_____

Prep your body to repair while you sleep
2 minute Nightly Visualization

Visualize running your goal run. Picture the scene moving by, feel the air around you and think about how it will feel as you powerfully and effortlessly glide through the run. Before you go to sleep, close your eyes for 1 minute and visualize running now.

Visualize cells in your body healing, repairing, making you stronger & rebuilding tissue. Before you go to sleep....
Close your eyes for 1 minute and visualize the healing now.

Morning Recovery Preparation Exercise DAY 10 Date:_____

My goal run is:

Once I can do that run, I will know I am recovered!

Visualize cells in your body healing, repairing, making you stronger & rebuilding tissue. Close your eyes for 1 minute and visualize the healing now.

Visualize running your goal run. Picture the scene moving by, feel the air around you and think about how it will feel as you powerfully and effortlessly glide through the run. Close your eyes for 1 minute and visualize running now.

Daily Pain Assessment:
Notice and write down any pain, stiffness or discomfort you feel this morning.
_____
_____
_____
_____

Recognize progress:
How have these uncomfortable feelings diminished or improved over the past week?
_____
_____
_____

Nutrition Plan to Fuel Today's Recovery. What/when will you eat/drink today:

Breakfast:_____ a.m.
Morning snack or mini-meal: _____ a.m.
Lunch: _____ p.m.
Afternoon snack or mini-meal:_____ p.m.
Dinner:_____ p.m.
Fluids:_____
Most of my antioxidants will come from: _____
Injury recovery specific supplements: _____

Active Recovery Plan to Fuel Today's Progress.
What will I commit to doing today to strengthen and support my one injured part?
Legs:_____
Core: _____
Upper body: _____
NO-Load Aerobic exercises: _____
Low-Load Aerobic exercises: _____
Stretching:_____
Massage: _____
Other: _____

Evening Recognizing Recovery Exercises

Today I supported and protected my injury so it can keep healing.
What did I do to protect my injury during today's activities?
_____
_____

Today I prepared my whole body, making it stronger so it can better support my injury. What exercises did I do today that will me stronger and increase my fitness?
_____
_____

Today I fueled my body with healing nutrients.
What did I eat and drink today that will help my tissues heal and grow while I sleep tonight?
_____
_____

Prep your body to repair while you sleep
2 minute Nightly Visualization

Visualize running your goal run. Picture the scene moving by, feel the air around you and think about how it will feel as you powerfully and effortlessly glide through the run. Before you go to sleep, close your eyes for 1 minute and visualize running now.

Visualize cells in your body healing, repairing, making you stronger & rebuilding tissue.
Before you go to sleep....
Close your eyes for 1 minute and visualize the healing now.

Morning Recovery Preparation Exercise DAY 11 Date:_____

My goal run is:

Once I can do that run, I will know I am recovered!

Visualize cells in your body healing, repairing, making you stronger & rebuilding tissue. Close your eyes for 1 minute and visualize the healing now.

Visualize running your goal run. Picture the scene moving by, feel the air around you and think about how it will feel as you powerfully and effortlessly glide through the run. Close your eyes for 1 minute and visualize running now.

Daily Pain Assessment:
Notice and write down any pain, stiffness or discomfort you feel this morning.
_____
_____
_____
_____

Recognize progress:
How have these uncomfortable feelings diminished or improved over the past week?
_____
_____
_____

Nutrition Plan to Fuel Today's Recovery. What/when will you eat/drink today:

Breakfast:_____ a.m.
Morning snack or mini-meal: _____ a.m.
Lunch: _____ p.m.
Afternoon snack or mini-meal:_____ p.m.
Dinner:_____ p.m.
Fluids:_____
Most of my antioxidants will come from: _____
Injury recovery specific supplements: _____

Active Recovery Plan to Fuel Today's Progress.
What will I commit to doing today to strengthen and support my one injured part?
Legs:_____
Core: _____
Upper body: _____
NO-Load Aerobic exercises: _____
Low-Load Aerobic exercises: _____
Stretching:_____
Massage: _____
Other: _____

Evening Recognizing Recovery Exercises

Today I supported and protected my injury so it can keep healing.
What did I do to protect my injury during today's activities?
_____
_____

Today I prepared my whole body, making it stronger so it can better support my injury. What exercises did I do today that will me stronger and increase my fitness?
_____
_____

Today I fueled my body with healing nutrients.
What did I eat and drink today that will help my tissues heal and grow while I sleep tonight?
_____
_____

Prep your body to repair while you sleep
2 minute Nightly Visualization

Visualize running your goal run. Picture the scene moving by, feel the air around you and think about how it will feel as you powerfully and effortlessly glide through the run.
Before you go to sleep, close your eyes for 1 minute and visualize running now.

Visualize cells in your body healing, repairing, making you stronger & rebuilding tissue.
Before you go to sleep....
Close your eyes for 1 minute and visualize the healing now.

Morning Recovery Preparation Exercise DAY 12 Date:_____

My goal run is:

Once I can do that run, I will know I am recovered!

Visualize cells in your body healing, repairing, making you stronger & rebuilding tissue. Close your eyes for 1 minute and visualize the healing now.

Visualize running your goal run. Picture the scene moving by, feel the air around you and think about how it will feel as you powerfully and effortlessly glide through the run. Close your eyes for 1 minute and visualize running now.

Daily Pain Assessment:
Notice and write down any pain, stiffness or discomfort you feel this morning.
_____
_____
_____
_____

Recognize progress:
How have these uncomfortable feelings diminished or improved over the past week?
_____
_____
_____

Nutrition Plan to Fuel Today's Recovery. What/when will you eat/drink today:

Breakfast:_____ a.m.
Morning snack or mini-meal: _____ a.m.
Lunch: _____ p.m.
Afternoon snack or mini-meal:_____ p.m.
Dinner:_____ p.m.
Fluids:_____
Most of my antioxidants will come from: _____
Injury recovery specific supplements: _____

Active Recovery Plan to Fuel Today's Progress.
What will I commit to doing today to strengthen and support my one injured part?
Legs: _____
Core: _____
Upper body: _____
NO-Load Aerobic exercises: _____
Low-Load Aerobic exercises: _____
Stretching: _____
Massage: _____
Other: _____

Evening Recognizing Recovery Exercises

Today I supported and protected my injury so it can keep healing.
What did I do to protect my injury during today's activities?
_____
_____

Today I prepared my whole body, making it stronger so it can better support my injury. What exercises did I do today that will me stronger and increase my fitness?
_____
_____

Today I fueled my body with healing nutrients.
What did I eat and drink today that will help my tissues heal and grow while I sleep tonight?
_____
_____

Prep your body to repair while you sleep
2 minute Nightly Visualization

Visualize running your goal run. Picture the scene moving by, feel the air around you and think about how it will feel as you powerfully and effortlessly glide through the run.
Before you go to sleep, close your eyes for 1 minute and visualize running now.

Visualize cells in your body healing, repairing, making you stronger & rebuilding tissue.
Before you go to sleep....
Close your eyes for 1 minute and visualize the healing now.

Morning Recovery Preparation Exercise DAY 13 Date:_____

My goal run is:

Once I can do that run, I will know I am recovered!

Visualize cells in your body healing, repairing, making you stronger & rebuilding tissue. Close your eyes for 1 minute and visualize the healing now.

Visualize running your goal run. Picture the scene moving by, feel the air around you and think about how it will feel as you powerfully and effortlessly glide through the run. Close your eyes for 1 minute and visualize running now.

Daily Pain Assessment:
Notice and write down any pain, stiffness or discomfort you feel this morning.
_____
_____
_____
_____

Recognize progress:
How have these uncomfortable feelings diminished or improved over the past week?
_____
_____
_____

Nutrition Plan to Fuel Today's Recovery. What/when will you eat/drink today:

Breakfast:_____ a.m.
Morning snack or mini-meal: _____ a.m.
Lunch: _____ p.m.
Afternoon snack or mini-meal:_____ p.m.
Dinner:_____ p.m.
Fluids:_____
Most of my antioxidants will come from: _____
Injury recovery specific supplements: _____

Active Recovery Plan to Fuel Today's Progress.
What will I commit to doing today to strengthen and support my one injured part?
Legs:_____
Core: _____
Upper body: _____
NO-Load Aerobic exercises: _____
Low-Load Aerobic exercises: _____
Stretching:_____
Massage: _____
Other: _____

Evening Recognizing Recovery Exercises

Today I supported and protected my injury so it can keep healing.
What did I do to protect my injury during today's activities?
_____
_____

Today I prepared my whole body, making it stronger so it can better support my injury. What exercises did I do today that will me stronger and increase my fitness?
_____
_____

Today I fueled my body with healing nutrients.
What did I eat and drink today that will help my tissues heal and grow while I sleep tonight?
_____
_____

Prep your body to repair while you sleep
2 minute Nightly Visualization

Visualize running your goal run. Picture the scene moving by, feel the air around you and think about how it will feel as you powerfully and effortlessly glide through the run. Before you go to sleep, close your eyes for 1 minute and visualize running now.

Visualize cells in your body healing, repairing, making you stronger & rebuilding tissue.
Before you go to sleep....
Close your eyes for 1 minute and visualize the healing now.

Morning Recovery Preparation Exercise DAY 14 Date:_____

My goal run is:

Once I can do that run, I will know I am recovered!

Visualize cells in your body healing, repairing, making you stronger & rebuilding tissue. Close your eyes for 1 minute and visualize the healing now.

Visualize running your goal run. Picture the scene moving by, feel the air around you and think about how it will feel as you powerfully and effortlessly glide through the run. Close your eyes for 1 minute and visualize running now.

Daily Pain Assessment:
Notice and write down any pain, stiffness or discomfort you feel this morning.
_____
_____
_____
_____

Recognize progress:
How have these uncomfortable feelings diminished or improved over the past week?
_____
_____
_____

Nutrition Plan to Fuel Today's Recovery. What/when will you eat/drink today:

Breakfast:_____ a.m.
Morning snack or mini-meal: _____ a.m.
Lunch: _____ p.m.
Afternoon snack or mini-meal:_____ p.m.
Dinner:_____ p.m.
Fluids:_____
Most of my antioxidants will come from: _____
Injury recovery specific supplements: _____

Active Recovery Plan to Fuel Today's Progress.
What will I commit to doing today to strengthen and support my one injured part?
Legs:_____
Core: _____
Upper body: _____
NO-Load Aerobic exercises: _____
Low-Load Aerobic exercises: _____
Stretching:_____
Massage: _____
Other: _____

Evening Recognizing Recovery Exercises

Today I supported and protected my injury so it can keep healing.
What did I do to protect my injury during today's activities?
_____
_____

Today I prepared my whole body, making it stronger so it can better support my injury. What exercises did I do today that will me stronger and increase my fitness?
_____
_____

Today I fueled my body with healing nutrients.
What did I eat and drink today that will help my tissues heal and grow while I sleep tonight?
_____
_____

Prep your body to repair while you sleep
2 minute Nightly Visualization

Visualize running your goal run. Picture the scene moving by, feel the air around you and think about how it will feel as you powerfully and effortlessly glide through the run.
Before you go to sleep, close your eyes for 1 minute and visualize running now.

Visualize cells in your body healing, repairing, making you stronger & rebuilding tissue.
Before you go to sleep....
Close your eyes for 1 minute and visualize the healing now.

Morning Recovery Preparation Exercise DAY 15 Date:_____

My goal run is:

                        Once I can do that run, I will know I am recovered!

Visualize cells in your body healing, repairing, making you stronger & rebuilding tissue. Close your eyes for 1 minute and visualize the healing now.

Visualize running your goal run. Picture the scene moving by, feel the air around you and think about how it will feel as you powerfully and effortlessly glide through the run. Close your eyes for 1 minute and visualize running now.

Daily Pain Assessment:
Notice and write down any pain, stiffness or discomfort you feel this morning.
_____
_____
_____
_____

Recognize progress:
How have these uncomfortable feelings diminished or improved over the past week?
_____
_____
_____

Nutrition Plan to Fuel Today's Recovery. What/when will you eat/drink today:

Breakfast:_____ a.m.
Morning snack or mini-meal: _____ a.m.
Lunch: _____ p.m.
Afternoon snack or mini-meal:_____ p.m.
Dinner:_____ p.m.
Fluids:_____
Most of my antioxidants will come from: _____
Injury recovery specific supplements: _____

Active Recovery Plan to Fuel Today's Progress.
What will I commit to doing today to strengthen and support my one injured part?
Legs:_____
Core: _____
Upper body: _____
NO-Load Aerobic exercises: _____
Low-Load Aerobic exercises: _____
Stretching:_____
Massage: _____
Other: _____

Evening Recognizing Recovery Exercises

Today I supported and protected my injury so it can keep healing.
What did I do to protect my injury during today's activities?
_____
_____

Today I prepared my whole body, making it stronger so it can better support my injury. What exercises did I do today that will me stronger and increase my fitness?
_____
_____

Today I fueled my body with healing nutrients.
What did I eat and drink today that will help my tissues heal and grow while I sleep tonight?
_____
_____

Prep your body to repair while you sleep
2 minute Nightly Visualization

Visualize running your goal run. Picture the scene moving by, feel the air around you and think about how it will feel as you powerfully and effortlessly glide through the run. Before you go to sleep, close your eyes for 1 minute and visualize running now.

Visualize cells in your body healing, repairing, making you stronger & rebuilding tissue.
Before you go to sleep....
Close your eyes for 1 minute and visualize the healing now.

Morning Recovery Preparation Exercise DAY 16 Date:_____

My goal run is:

Once I can do that run, I will know I am recovered!

Visualize cells in your body healing, repairing, making you stronger & rebuilding tissue. Close your eyes for 1 minute and visualize the healing now.

Visualize running your goal run. Picture the scene moving by, feel the air around you and think about how it will feel as you powerfully and effortlessly glide through the run. Close your eyes for 1 minute and visualize running now.

Daily Pain Assessment:
Notice and write down any pain, stiffness or discomfort you feel this morning.
_____
_____
_____
_____

Recognize progress:
How have these uncomfortable feelings diminished or improved over the past week?
_____
_____
_____

Nutrition Plan to Fuel Today's Recovery. What/when will you eat/drink today:

Breakfast:_____ a.m.
Morning snack or mini-meal: _____ a.m.
Lunch: _____ p.m.
Afternoon snack or mini-meal:_____ p.m.
Dinner:_____ p.m.
Fluids:_____
Most of my antioxidants will come from: _____
Injury recovery specific supplements: _____

Active Recovery Plan to Fuel Today's Progress.
What will I commit to doing today to strengthen and support my one injured part?
Legs:_____
Core: _____
Upper body: _____
NO-Load Aerobic exercises: _____
Low-Load Aerobic exercises: _____
Stretching:_____
Massage: _____
Other: _____

Evening Recognizing Recovery Exercises

Today I supported and protected my injury so it can keep healing.
What did I do to protect my injury during today's activities?
_____
_____

Today I prepared my whole body, making it stronger so it can better support my injury. What exercises did I do today that will me stronger and increase my fitness?
_____
_____

Today I fueled my body with healing nutrients.
What did I eat and drink today that will help my tissues heal and grow while I sleep tonight?
_____
_____

Prep your body to repair while you sleep
2 minute Nightly Visualization

Visualize running your goal run. Picture the scene moving by, feel the air around you and think about how it will feel as you powerfully and effortlessly glide through the run.
Before you go to sleep, close your eyes for 1 minute and visualize running now.

Visualize cells in your body healing, repairing, making you stronger & rebuilding tissue.
Before you go to sleep….
Close your eyes for 1 minute and visualize the healing now.

Morning Recovery Preparation Exercise DAY 17 Date:_____

My goal run is:

Once I can do that run, I will know I am recovered!

Visualize cells in your body healing, repairing, making you stronger & rebuilding tissue. Close your eyes for 1 minute and visualize the healing now.

Visualize running your goal run. Picture the scene moving by, feel the air around you and think about how it will feel as you powerfully and effortlessly glide through the run. Close your eyes for 1 minute and visualize running now.

Daily Pain Assessment:
Notice and write down any pain, stiffness or discomfort you feel this morning.
_____
_____
_____
_____

Recognize progress:
How have these uncomfortable feelings diminished or improved over the past week?
_____
_____
_____

Nutrition Plan to Fuel Today's Recovery. What/when will you eat/drink today:

Breakfast:_____ a.m.
Morning snack or mini-meal: _____ a.m.
Lunch: _____ p.m.
Afternoon snack or mini-meal:_____ p.m.
Dinner:_____ p.m.
Fluids:_____
Most of my antioxidants will come from: _____
Injury recovery specific supplements: _____

Active Recovery Plan to Fuel Today's Progress.
What will I commit to doing today to strengthen and support my one injured part?
Legs:_____
Core: _____
Upper body: _____
NO-Load Aerobic exercises: _____
Low-Load Aerobic exercises: _____
Stretching:_____
Massage: _____
Other: _____

Evening Recognizing Recovery Exercises

Today I supported and protected my injury so it can keep healing.
What did I do to protect my injury during today's activities?
_____
_____

Today I prepared my whole body, making it stronger so it can better support my injury. What exercises did I do today that will me stronger and increase my fitness?
_____
_____

Today I fueled my body with healing nutrients.
What did I eat and drink today that will help my tissues heal and grow while I sleep tonight?
_____
_____

Prep your body to repair while you sleep
2 minute Nightly Visualization

Visualize running your goal run. Picture the scene moving by, feel the air around you and think about how it will feel as you powerfully and effortlessly glide through the run.
Before you go to sleep, close your eyes for 1 minute and visualize running now.

Visualize cells in your body healing, repairing, making you stronger & rebuilding tissue.
Before you go to sleep....
Close your eyes for 1 minute and visualize the healing now.

Morning Recovery Preparation Exercise DAY 18 Date:_____

My goal run is:

Once I can do that run, I will know I am recovered!

Visualize cells in your body healing, repairing, making you stronger & rebuilding tissue. Close your eyes for 1 minute and visualize the healing now.

Visualize running your goal run. Picture the scene moving by, feel the air around you and think about how it will feel as you powerfully and effortlessly glide through the run. Close your eyes for 1 minute and visualize running now.

Daily Pain Assessment:
Notice and write down any pain, stiffness or discomfort you feel this morning.
_____
_____
_____
_____

Recognize progress:
How have these uncomfortable feelings diminished or improved over the past week?
_____
_____
_____

Nutrition Plan to Fuel Today's Recovery. What/when will you eat/drink today:

Breakfast:_____ a.m.
Morning snack or mini-meal: _____ a.m.
Lunch: _____ p.m.
Afternoon snack or mini-meal:_____ p.m.
Dinner:_____ p.m.
Fluids:_____
Most of my antioxidants will come from: _____
Injury recovery specific supplements: _____

Active Recovery Plan to Fuel Today's Progress.
What will I commit to doing today to strengthen and support my one injured part?
Legs: _____
Core: _____
Upper body: _____
NO-Load Aerobic exercises: _____
Low-Load Aerobic exercises: _____
Stretching: _____
Massage: _____
Other: _____

Evening Recognizing Recovery Exercises

Today I supported and protected my injury so it can keep healing.
What did I do to protect my injury during today's activities?
_____
_____

Today I prepared my whole body, making it stronger so it can better support my injury. What exercises did I do today that will me stronger and increase my fitness?
_____
_____

Today I fueled my body with healing nutrients.
What did I eat and drink today that will help my tissues heal and grow while I sleep tonight?
_____
_____

Prep your body to repair while you sleep
2 minute Nightly Visualization

Visualize running your goal run. Picture the scene moving by, feel the air around you and think about how it will feel as you powerfully and effortlessly glide through the run.
Before you go to sleep, close your eyes for 1 minute and visualize running now.

Visualize cells in your body healing, repairing, making you stronger & rebuilding tissue.
Before you go to sleep….
Close your eyes for 1 minute and visualize the healing now.

Morning Recovery Preparation Exercise DAY 19 Date:_____

My goal run is:

Once I can do that run, I will know I am recovered!

Visualize cells in your body healing, repairing, making you stronger & rebuilding tissue. Close your eyes for 1 minute and visualize the healing now.

Visualize running your goal run. Picture the scene moving by, feel the air around you and think about how it will feel as you powerfully and effortlessly glide through the run. Close your eyes for 1 minute and visualize running now.

Daily Pain Assessment:
Notice and write down any pain, stiffness or discomfort you feel this morning.
_____
_____
_____
_____

Recognize progress:
How have these uncomfortable feelings diminished or improved over the past week?
_____
_____
_____

Nutrition Plan to Fuel Today's Recovery. What/when will you eat/drink today:

Breakfast:_____ a.m.
Morning snack or mini-meal: _____ a.m.
Lunch: _____ p.m.
Afternoon snack or mini-meal:_____ p.m.
Dinner:_____ p.m.
Fluids:_____
Most of my antioxidants will come from: _____
Injury recovery specific supplements: _____

Active Recovery Plan to Fuel Today's Progress.
What will I commit to doing today to strengthen and support my one injured part?
Legs:_____
Core: _____
Upper body: _____
NO-Load Aerobic exercises: _____
Low-Load Aerobic exercises: _____
Stretching:_____
Massage: _____
Other: _____

Evening Recognizing Recovery Exercises

Today I supported and protected my injury so it can keep healing.
What did I do to protect my injury during today's activities?
_____
_____

Today I prepared my whole body, making it stronger so it can better support my injury. What exercises did I do today that will me stronger and increase my fitness?
_____
_____

Today I fueled my body with healing nutrients.
What did I eat and drink today that will help my tissues heal and grow while I sleep tonight?
_____
_____

Prep your body to repair while you sleep
2 minute Nightly Visualization

Visualize running your goal run. Picture the scene moving by, feel the air around you and think about how it will feel as you powerfully and effortlessly glide through the run.
Before you go to sleep, close your eyes for 1 minute and visualize running now.

Visualize cells in your body healing, repairing, making you stronger & rebuilding tissue.
Before you go to sleep....
Close your eyes for 1 minute and visualize the healing now.

Morning Recovery Preparation Exercise DAY 20 Date:_____

My goal run is:

Once I can do that run, I will know I am recovered!

Visualize cells in your body healing, repairing, making you stronger & rebuilding tissue. Close your eyes for 1 minute and visualize the healing now.

Visualize running your goal run. Picture the scene moving by, feel the air around you and think about how it will feel as you powerfully and effortlessly glide through the run. Close your eyes for 1 minute and visualize running now.

Daily Pain Assessment:
Notice and write down any pain, stiffness or discomfort you feel this morning.
_____
_____
_____
_____

Recognize progress:
How have these uncomfortable feelings diminished or improved over the past week?
_____
_____
_____

Nutrition Plan to Fuel Today's Recovery. What/when will you eat/drink today:

Breakfast:_____ a.m.
Morning snack or mini-meal: _____ a.m.
Lunch: _____ p.m.
Afternoon snack or mini-meal:_____ p.m.
Dinner:_____ p.m.
Fluids:_____
Most of my antioxidants will come from: _____
Injury recovery specific supplements: _____

Active Recovery Plan to Fuel Today's Progress.
What will I commit to doing today to strengthen and support my one injured part?
Legs:_____
Core: _____
Upper body: _____
NO-Load Aerobic exercises: _____
Low-Load Aerobic exercises: _____
Stretching:_____
Massage: _____
Other: _____

Evening Recognizing Recovery Exercises

Today I supported and protected my injury so it can keep healing.
What did I do to protect my injury during today's activities?
_____
_____

Today I prepared my whole body, making it stronger so it can better support my injury. What exercises did I do today that will me stronger and increase my fitness?
_____
_____

Today I fueled my body with healing nutrients.
What did I eat and drink today that will help my tissues heal and grow while I sleep tonight?
_____
_____

Prep your body to repair while you sleep
2 minute Nightly Visualization

Visualize running your goal run. Picture the scene moving by, feel the air around you and think about how it will feel as you powerfully and effortlessly glide through the run.
Before you go to sleep, close your eyes for 1 minute and visualize running now.

Visualize cells in your body healing, repairing, making you stronger & rebuilding tissue.
Before you go to sleep….
Close your eyes for 1 minute and visualize the healing now.

Morning Recovery Preparation Exercise DAY 21 Date:_____

My goal run is:

Once I can do that run, I will know I am recovered!

Visualize cells in your body healing, repairing, making you stronger & rebuilding tissue. Close your eyes for 1 minute and visualize the healing now.

Visualize running your goal run. Picture the scene moving by, feel the air around you and think about how it will feel as you powerfully and effortlessly glide through the run. Close your eyes for 1 minute and visualize running now.

Daily Pain Assessment:
Notice and write down any pain, stiffness or discomfort you feel this morning.
_____
_____
_____
_____

Recognize progress:
How have these uncomfortable feelings diminished or improved over the past week?
_____
_____
_____

Nutrition Plan to Fuel Today's Recovery. What/when will you eat/drink today:

Breakfast:_____ a.m.
Morning snack or mini-meal: _____ a.m.
Lunch: _____ p.m.
Afternoon snack or mini-meal:_____ p.m.
Dinner:_____ p.m.
Fluids:_____
Most of my antioxidants will come from: _____
Injury recovery specific supplements: _____

Active Recovery Plan to Fuel Today's Progress.
What will I commit to doing today to strengthen and support my one injured part?
Legs:_____
Core: _____
Upper body: _____
NO-Load Aerobic exercises: _____
Low-Load Aerobic exercises: _____
Stretching:_____
Massage: _____
Other: _____

Evening Recognizing Recovery Exercises

Today I supported and protected my injury so it can keep healing.
What did I do to protect my injury during today's activities?
_____
_____

Today I prepared my whole body, making it stronger so it can better support my injury. What exercises did I do today that will me stronger and increase my fitness?
_____
_____

Today I fueled my body with healing nutrients.
What did I eat and drink today that will help my tissues heal and grow while I sleep tonight?
_____
_____

Prep your body to repair while you sleep
2 minute Nightly Visualization

Visualize running your goal run. Picture the scene moving by, feel the air around you and think about how it will feel as you powerfully and effortlessly glide through the run. Before you go to sleep, close your eyes for 1 minute and visualize running now.

Visualize cells in your body healing, repairing, making you stronger & rebuilding tissue.
Before you go to sleep....
Close your eyes for 1 minute and visualize the healing now.

Morning Recovery Preparation Exercise DAY 22 Date:_____

My goal run is:

Once I can do that run, I will know I am recovered!

Visualize cells in your body healing, repairing, making you stronger & rebuilding tissue. Close your eyes for 1 minute and visualize the healing now.

Visualize running your goal run. Picture the scene moving by, feel the air around you and think about how it will feel as you powerfully and effortlessly glide through the run. Close your eyes for 1 minute and visualize running now.

Daily Pain Assessment:
Notice and write down any pain, stiffness or discomfort you feel this morning.
_____
_____
_____
_____

Recognize progress:
How have these uncomfortable feelings diminished or improved over the past week?
_____
_____
_____

Nutrition Plan to Fuel Today's Recovery. What/when will you eat/drink today:

Breakfast:_____ a.m.
Morning snack or mini-meal: _____ a.m.
Lunch: _____ p.m.
Afternoon snack or mini-meal:_____ p.m.
Dinner:_____ p.m.
Fluids:_____
Most of my antioxidants will come from: _____
Injury recovery specific supplements: _____

Active Recovery Plan to Fuel Today's Progress.
What will I commit to doing today to strengthen and support my one injured part?
Legs:_____
Core: _____
Upper body: _____
NO-Load Aerobic exercises: _____
Low-Load Aerobic exercises: _____
Stretching:_____
Massage: _____
Other: _____

Evening Recognizing Recovery Exercises

Today I supported and protected my injury so it can keep healing.
What did I do to protect my injury during today's activities?
_____
_____

Today I prepared my whole body, making it stronger so it can better support my injury. What exercises did I do today that will me stronger and increase my fitness?
_____
_____

Today I fueled my body with healing nutrients.
What did I eat and drink today that will help my tissues heal and grow while I sleep tonight?
_____
_____

Prep your body to repair while you sleep
2 minute Nightly Visualization

Visualize running your goal run. Picture the scene moving by, feel the air around you and think about how it will feel as you powerfully and effortlessly glide through the run.
Before you go to sleep, close your eyes for 1 minute and visualize running now.

Visualize cells in your body healing, repairing, making you stronger & rebuilding tissue.
Before you go to sleep….
Close your eyes for 1 minute and visualize the healing now.

Morning Recovery Preparation Exercise DAY 23 Date:_____

My goal run is:

Once I can do that run, I will know I am recovered!

Visualize cells in your body healing, repairing, making you stronger & rebuilding tissue. Close your eyes for 1 minute and visualize the healing now.

Visualize running your goal run. Picture the scene moving by, feel the air around you and think about how it will feel as you powerfully and effortlessly glide through the run. Close your eyes for 1 minute and visualize running now.

Daily Pain Assessment:
Notice and write down any pain, stiffness or discomfort you feel this morning.
_____
_____
_____
_____

Recognize progress:
How have these uncomfortable feelings diminished or improved over the past week?
_____
_____
_____

Nutrition Plan to Fuel Today's Recovery. What/when will you eat/drink today:

Breakfast:_____
Morning snack or mini-meal: _____ a.m.
Lunch: _____ a.m.
Afternoon snack or mini-meal:_____ p.m.
Dinner:_____ p.m.
Fluids:_____ p.m.
Most of my antioxidants will come from: _____
Injury recovery specific supplements: _____

Active Recovery Plan to Fuel Today's Progress.
What will I commit to doing today to strengthen and support my one injured part?
Legs:_____
Core: _____
Upper body: _____
NO-Load Aerobic exercises: _____
Low-Load Aerobic exercises: _____
Stretching:_____
Massage: _____
Other: _____

Evening Recognizing Recovery Exercises

Today I supported and protected my injury so it can keep healing.
What did I do to protect my injury during today's activities?
_____
_____

Today I prepared my whole body, making it stronger so it can better support my injury. What exercises did I do today that will me stronger and increase my fitness?
_____
_____

Today I fueled my body with healing nutrients.
What did I eat and drink today that will help my tissues heal and grow while I sleep tonight?
_____
_____

Prep your body to repair while you sleep
2 minute Nightly Visualization

Visualize running your goal run. Picture the scene moving by, feel the air around you and think about how it will feel as you powerfully and effortlessly glide through the run.
Before you go to sleep, close your eyes for 1 minute and visualize running now.

Visualize cells in your body healing, repairing, making you stronger & rebuilding tissue.
Before you go to sleep....
Close your eyes for 1 minute and visualize the healing now.

Morning Recovery Preparation Exercise DAY 24 Date:_____

My goal run is:

Once I can do that run, I will know I am recovered!

Visualize cells in your body healing, repairing, making you stronger & rebuilding tissue. Close your eyes for 1 minute and visualize the healing now.

Visualize running your goal run. Picture the scene moving by, feel the air around you and think about how it will feel as you powerfully and effortlessly glide through the run. Close your eyes for 1 minute and visualize running now.

Daily Pain Assessment:
Notice and write down any pain, stiffness or discomfort you feel this morning.
_____
_____
_____
_____

Recognize progress:
How have these uncomfortable feelings diminished or improved over the past week?
_____
_____
_____

Nutrition Plan to Fuel Today's Recovery. What/when will you eat/drink today:

Breakfast:_____ a.m.
Morning snack or mini-meal: _____ a.m.
Lunch: _____ p.m.
Afternoon snack or mini-meal:_____ p.m.
Dinner:_____ p.m.
Fluids:_____
Most of my antioxidants will come from: _____
Injury recovery specific supplements: _____

Active Recovery Plan to Fuel Today's Progress.
What will I commit to doing today to strengthen and support my one injured part?
Legs:_____
Core: _____
Upper body: _____
NO-Load Aerobic exercises: _____
Low-Load Aerobic exercises: _____
Stretching:_____
Massage: _____
Other: _____

Evening Recognizing Recovery Exercises

Today I supported and protected my injury so it can keep healing.
What did I do to protect my injury during today's activities?
_____
_____

Today I prepared my whole body, making it stronger so it can better support my injury. What exercises did I do today that will me stronger and increase my fitness?
_____
_____

Today I fueled my body with healing nutrients.
What did I eat and drink today that will help my tissues heal and grow while I sleep tonight?
_____
_____

Prep your body to repair while you sleep
2 minute Nightly Visualization

Visualize running your goal run. Picture the scene moving by, feel the air around you and think about how it will feel as you powerfully and effortlessly glide through the run.
Before you go to sleep, close your eyes for 1 minute and visualize running now.

Visualize cells in your body healing, repairing, making you stronger & rebuilding tissue.
Before you go to sleep….
Close your eyes for 1 minute and visualize the healing now.

Morning Recovery Preparation Exercise DAY 25 Date:_____

My goal run is:

                                   Once I can do that run, I will know I am recovered!

Visualize cells in your body healing, repairing, making you stronger & rebuilding tissue. Close your eyes for 1 minute and visualize the healing now.

Visualize running your goal run. Picture the scene moving by, feel the air around you and think about how it will feel as you powerfully and effortlessly glide through the run. Close your eyes for 1 minute and visualize running now.

Daily Pain Assessment:
Notice and write down any pain, stiffness or discomfort you feel this morning.
_____
_____
_____
_____

Recognize progress:
How have these uncomfortable feelings diminished or improved over the past week?
_____
_____
_____

Nutrition Plan to Fuel Today's Recovery. What/when will you eat/drink today:

Breakfast:_____ a.m.
Morning snack or mini-meal: _____ a.m.
Lunch: _____ p.m.
Afternoon snack or mini-meal:_____ p.m.
Dinner:_____ p.m.
Fluids:_____
Most of my antioxidants will come from: _____
Injury recovery specific supplements: _____

Active Recovery Plan to Fuel Today's Progress.
What will I commit to doing today to strengthen and support my one injured part?
Legs:_____
Core: _____
Upper body: _____
NO-Load Aerobic exercises: _____
Low-Load Aerobic exercises: _____
Stretching:_____
Massage: _____
Other: _____

Evening Recognizing Recovery Exercises

Today I supported and protected my injury so it can keep healing.
What did I do to protect my injury during today's activities?
_____
_____

Today I prepared my whole body, making it stronger so it can better support my injury. What exercises did I do today that will me stronger and increase my fitness?
_____
_____

Today I fueled my body with healing nutrients.
What did I eat and drink today that will help my tissues heal and grow while I sleep tonight?
_____
_____

Prep your body to repair while you sleep
2 minute Nightly Visualization

Visualize running your goal run. Picture the scene moving by, feel the air around you and think about how it will feel as you powerfully and effortlessly glide through the run. Before you go to sleep, close your eyes for 1 minute and visualize running now.

Visualize cells in your body healing, repairing, making you stronger & rebuilding tissue. Before you go to sleep....
Close your eyes for 1 minute and visualize the healing now.

Morning Recovery Preparation Exercise DAY 26 Date:_____

My goal run is:

Once I can do that run, I will know I am recovered!

Visualize cells in your body healing, repairing, making you stronger & rebuilding tissue. Close your eyes for 1 minute and visualize the healing now.

Visualize running your goal run. Picture the scene moving by, feel the air around you and think about how it will feel as you powerfully and effortlessly glide through the run. Close your eyes for 1 minute and visualize running now.

Daily Pain Assessment:
Notice and write down any pain, stiffness or discomfort you feel this morning.
_____
_____
_____
_____

Recognize progress:
How have these uncomfortable feelings diminished or improved over the past week?
_____
_____
_____

Nutrition Plan to Fuel Today's Recovery. What/when will you eat/drink today:

Breakfast:_____ a.m.
Morning snack or mini-meal: _____ a.m.
Lunch: _____ p.m.
Afternoon snack or mini-meal:_____ p.m.
Dinner:_____ p.m.
Fluids:_____
Most of my antioxidants will come from: _____
Injury recovery specific supplements: _____

Active Recovery Plan to Fuel Today's Progress.
What will I commit to doing today to strengthen and support my one injured part?
Legs:_____
Core: _____
Upper body: _____
NO-Load Aerobic exercises: _____
Low-Load Aerobic exercises: _____
Stretching:_____
Massage: _____
Other: _____

Evening Recognizing Recovery Exercises

Today I supported and protected my injury so it can keep healing.
What did I do to protect my injury during today's activities?
_____
_____

Today I prepared my whole body, making it stronger so it can better support my injury. What exercises did I do today that will me stronger and increase my fitness?
_____
_____

Today I fueled my body with healing nutrients.
What did I eat and drink today that will help my tissues heal and grow while I sleep tonight?
_____
_____

Prep your body to repair while you sleep
2 minute Nightly Visualization

Visualize running your goal run. Picture the scene moving by, feel the air around you and think about how it will feel as you powerfully and effortlessly glide through the run.
Before you go to sleep, close your eyes for 1 minute and visualize running now.

Visualize cells in your body healing, repairing, making you stronger & rebuilding tissue.
Before you go to sleep....
Close your eyes for 1 minute and visualize the healing now.

Morning Recovery Preparation Exercise DAY 27 Date:_____

My goal run is:

Once I can do that run, I will know I am recovered!

Visualize cells in your body healing, repairing, making you stronger & rebuilding tissue. Close your eyes for 1 minute and visualize the healing now.

Visualize running your goal run. Picture the scene moving by, feel the air around you and think about how it will feel as you powerfully and effortlessly glide through the run. Close your eyes for 1 minute and visualize running now.

Daily Pain Assessment:
Notice and write down any pain, stiffness or discomfort you feel this morning.
_____
_____
_____
_____

Recognize progress:
How have these uncomfortable feelings diminished or improved over the past week?
_____
_____
_____

Nutrition Plan to Fuel Today's Recovery. What/when will you eat/drink today:

Breakfast:_____ a.m.
Morning snack or mini-meal: _____ a.m.
Lunch: _____ p.m.
Afternoon snack or mini-meal:_____ p.m.
Dinner:_____ p.m.
Fluids:_____
Most of my antioxidants will come from: _____
Injury recovery specific supplements: _____

Active Recovery Plan to Fuel Today's Progress.
What will I commit to doing today to strengthen and support my one injured part?
Legs:_____
Core: _____
Upper body: _____
NO-Load Aerobic exercises: _____
Low-Load Aerobic exercises: _____
Stretching:_____
Massage: _____
Other: _____

Evening Recognizing Recovery Exercises

Today I supported and protected my injury so it can keep healing.
What did I do to protect my injury during today's activities?
_____
_____

Today I prepared my whole body, making it stronger so it can better support my injury. What exercises did I do today that will me stronger and increase my fitness?
_____
_____

Today I fueled my body with healing nutrients.
What did I eat and drink today that will help my tissues heal and grow while I sleep tonight?
_____
_____

Prep your body to repair while you sleep
2 minute Nightly Visualization

Visualize running your goal run. Picture the scene moving by, feel the air around you and think about how it will feel as you powerfully and effortlessly glide through the run.
Before you go to sleep, close your eyes for 1 minute and visualize running now.

Visualize cells in your body healing, repairing, making you stronger & rebuilding tissue.
Before you go to sleep....
Close your eyes for 1 minute and visualize the healing now.

Morning Recovery Preparation Exercise DAY 28 Date:_____

My goal run is:

Once I can do that run, I will know I am recovered!

Visualize cells in your body healing, repairing, making you stronger & rebuilding tissue. Close your eyes for 1 minute and visualize the healing now.

Visualize running your goal run. Picture the scene moving by, feel the air around you and think about how it will feel as you powerfully and effortlessly glide through the run. Close your eyes for 1 minute and visualize running now.

Daily Pain Assessment:
Notice and write down any pain, stiffness or discomfort you feel this morning.
_____
_____
_____
_____

Recognize progress:
How have these uncomfortable feelings diminished or improved over the past week?
_____
_____
_____

Nutrition Plan to Fuel Today's Recovery. What/when will you eat/drink today:

Breakfast:_____ a.m.
Morning snack or mini-meal: _____ a.m.
Lunch: _____ p.m.
Afternoon snack or mini-meal:_____ p.m.
Dinner:_____ p.m.
Fluids:_____
Most of my antioxidants will come from: _____
Injury recovery specific supplements: _____

Active Recovery Plan to Fuel Today's Progress.
What will I commit to doing today to strengthen and support my one injured part?
Legs:_____
Core: _____
Upper body: _____
NO-Load Aerobic exercises: _____
Low-Load Aerobic exercises: _____
Stretching:_____
Massage: _____
Other: _____

Evening Recognizing Recovery Exercises

Today I supported and protected my injury so it can keep healing.
What did I do to protect my injury during today's activities?
_____
_____

Today I prepared my whole body, making it stronger so it can better support my injury. What exercises did I do today that will me stronger and increase my fitness?
_____
_____

Today I fueled my body with healing nutrients.
What did I eat and drink today that will help my tissues heal and grow while I sleep tonight?
_____
_____

Prep your body to repair while you sleep
2 minute Nightly Visualization

Visualize running your goal run. Picture the scene moving by, feel the air around you and think about how it will feel as you powerfully and effortlessly glide through the run.
Before you go to sleep, close your eyes for 1 minute and visualize running now.

Visualize cells in your body healing, repairing, making you stronger & rebuilding tissue.
Before you go to sleep....
Close your eyes for 1 minute and visualize the healing now.

Morning Recovery Preparation Exercise DAY 29 Date:_____

My goal run is:

Once I can do that run, I will know I am recovered!

Visualize cells in your body healing, repairing, making you stronger & rebuilding tissue. Close your eyes for 1 minute and visualize the healing now.

Visualize running your goal run. Picture the scene moving by, feel the air around you and think about how it will feel as you powerfully and effortlessly glide through the run. Close your eyes for 1 minute and visualize running now.

Daily Pain Assessment:
Notice and write down any pain, stiffness or discomfort you feel this morning.
_____
_____
_____
_____

Recognize progress:
How have these uncomfortable feelings diminished or improved over the past week?
_____
_____
_____

Nutrition Plan to Fuel Today's Recovery. What/when will you eat/drink today:

Breakfast:_____ a.m.
Morning snack or mini-meal: _____ a.m.
Lunch: _____ p.m.
Afternoon snack or mini-meal:_____ p.m.
Dinner:_____ p.m.
Fluids:_____
Most of my antioxidants will come from: _____
Injury recovery specific supplements: _____

Active Recovery Plan to Fuel Today's Progress.
What will I commit to doing today to strengthen and support my one injured part?
Legs:_____
Core: _____
Upper body: _____
NO-Load Aerobic exercises: _____
Low-Load Aerobic exercises: _____
Stretching:_____
Massage: _____
Other: _____

Evening Recognizing Recovery Exercises

Today I supported and protected my injury so it can keep healing.
What did I do to protect my injury during today's activities?
_____
_____

Today I prepared my whole body, making it stronger so it can better support my injury. What exercises did I do today that will me stronger and increase my fitness?
_____
_____

Today I fueled my body with healing nutrients.
What did I eat and drink today that will help my tissues heal and grow while I sleep tonight?
_____
_____

Prep your body to repair while you sleep
2 minute Nightly Visualization

Visualize running your goal run. Picture the scene moving by, feel the air around you and think about how it will feel as you powerfully and effortlessly glide through the run.
Before you go to sleep, close your eyes for 1 minute and visualize running now.

Visualize cells in your body healing, repairing, making you stronger & rebuilding tissue.
Before you go to sleep....
Close your eyes for 1 minute and visualize the healing now.

Morning Recovery Preparation Exercise DAY 30 Date:_____

My goal run is:

Once I can do that run, I will know I am recovered!

Visualize cells in your body healing, repairing, making you stronger & rebuilding tissue. Close your eyes for 1 minute and visualize the healing now.

Visualize running your goal run. Picture the scene moving by, feel the air around you and think about how it will feel as you powerfully and effortlessly glide through the run. Close your eyes for 1 minute and visualize running now.

Daily Pain Assessment:
Notice and write down any pain, stiffness or discomfort you feel this morning.
_____
_____
_____
_____

Recognize progress:
How have these uncomfortable feelings diminished or improved over the past week?
_____
_____
_____

Nutrition Plan to Fuel Today's Recovery. What/when will you eat/drink today:

Breakfast:_____ a.m.
Morning snack or mini-meal: _____ a.m.
Lunch: _____ p.m.
Afternoon snack or mini-meal:_____ p.m.
Dinner:_____ p.m.
Fluids:_____
Most of my antioxidants will come from: _____
Injury recovery specific supplements: _____

Active Recovery Plan to Fuel Today's Progress.
What will I commit to doing today to strengthen and support my one injured part?
Legs:_____
Core: _____
Upper body: _____
NO-Load Aerobic exercises: _____
Low-Load Aerobic exercises: _____
Stretching:_____
Massage: _____
Other: _____

Evening Recognizing Recovery Exercises

Today I supported and protected my injury so it can keep healing.
What did I do to protect my injury during today's activities?
_____
_____

Today I prepared my whole body, making it stronger so it can better support my injury. What exercises did I do today that will me stronger and increase my fitness?
_____
_____

Today I fueled my body with healing nutrients.
What did I eat and drink today that will help my tissues heal and grow while I sleep tonight?
_____
_____

Prep your body to repair while you sleep
2 minute Nightly Visualization

Visualize running your goal run. Picture the scene moving by, feel the air around you and think about how it will feel as you powerfully and effortlessly glide through the run. Before you go to sleep, close your eyes for 1 minute and visualize running now.

Visualize cells in your body healing, repairing, making you stronger & rebuilding tissue.
Before you go to sleep....
Close your eyes for 1 minute and visualize the healing now.

Appendix 1
Runner's
Pain Journal

Pain is a part of running. There is a saying often lauded by athletes and we have all heard, "Pain is just weakness leaving your body." We affectionately call our training studios "Pain Caves." We bask in the discomfort of pain, knowing it will make us stronger. In training we embrace pain as an ally.

But when you get an over-training injury, pain when running is no longer your friend. The pain forces you to run slower or run shorter distances. Pain forces you to skip workouts. Pain is wrecking your training schedule. Pain is in the way. Pain is your enemy.

In thinking about this, another saying comes to mind, "Keep your friends close, but keep your enemies closer." You can keep track of that pain and use it as a tool to recover as fast as possible and get back to running.

The Bad News:
Runners have a higher pain threshold.

A few years ago there was a research study published in the medical journal Pain[1]. The study systematically reviewed differences in pain perception between athletes and normally active people. The researchers report revealed that athletes possessed higher pain tolerance. The data from the meta-analysis suggest that regular physical activity is associated with specific alterations in pain perception.

So the bad news as an injured athlete is that you may be prone to ignoring pain as a warning sign. You may be at higher risk of hurting yourself, prolonging the injury and slowing your recovery since, as an athlete, you have a higher pain tolerance.

The Good News:
Runners have a higher level of somatic awareness.

All of that work you put into developing good running form, feeling for rates of intensity, noticing and charting levels of perceived exertion, all of that leads to what we call "somatic awareness." Simply put, runners like you have the ability to tell what's going on in your body. You can feel when your form is right. You can sense a sluggishness when you are having an "off day." You can sense muscular tightness.

When you get injured you really only have 3 signs of worsening injury: Pain, Swelling and Bruising. Pain is the easiest and most informative of all these signs. Pain tells you something is wrong and may indicate you are doing damage. Pain is dynamic. Pain can give you immediate feed-back and can be extremely useful.

A pain journal helps you map progress.

A few years ago I interviewed James Lawrence the IronCowboy. One of the most memorable moments in that episode was when he explained how some of the athlete he coaches will ask if they should start some new fad diet. His advice is always…keep a food journal first. You have to know what you are eating first. You have to understand where you are and then make changes that move you from that starting point to your ultimate destination.

A pain journal helps you convince yourself that you are getting better.

The same way a training schedule helps you recognize progress, see that you are realizing your goals, mapping your recovery with a pain journal can help you see trends and note progress. Since an injury is so stressful, you need to be able to see improvement. A positive outlook that comes from documented improvement will help you maintain a positive outlook and help you look for the light at the end of the tunnel, even when that light seems faint.

A pain journal helps your doctor decide how to customize your treatment plan and direct your recovery. A pain journal helps you decide when it is safe to run and how much you can advance your activity level or increase running distance.

If you are keeping a pain journal, don't take pain relievers. They can skew the results by masking pain. Just this week a runner called me for a second opinion. I actually thought she had a different problem than she had been told. I told her to stop taking the anti-inflammatories and her pain came back. So the anti-inflammatories were just masking her pain. The boot wasn't really fixing anything. It just seemed like she was getting better from the boot, when really it was just the pain medicine covering up the pain. So that's rule #1: compare apples to apples and do not take pain medicine while keeping a pain journal.

How to Use the Runner's Pain Journal.

Here is what you need to record in your pain journal:

Date. Most injured runners seem to be poor historians. We often have pain longer than we want to admit. Log the date so you really know when things happen.

Run distance. How far did you run? How many miles and where; track, street, soft jogging path or on a treadmill?

Run Intensity. How hard an effort was it? Rate the exercise session on a scale of 1-10.

Pain Location. Where exactly was the pain? Is the pain on the top of foot, ball of foot, heel, arch, Achilles, ankle, shin? Sometimes it changes. Write it down. Create a record. Put your finger on the most tender spot and take a picture of it.

Pain during your run. How much did it hurt? Log your perceived pain level during the run on a scale of 1 to 10.

Did it get better, worse, or stay the same throughout the run?

Did your pain go away during the run? If so, make a note of how many miles into the run, at what distance the pain went away.

If the pain went away during the run, did it come back again? If so, make a note of how many miles into the run, at what distance the pain came back.

What about later in the day? Did you have any pain or soreness later in the evening after your workout? If so, rate it on a scale of 1 to 10.

What about the next morning? Did you have any pain or soreness when you woke up and got out of bed the morning following your workout? If so, rate it on a scale of 1 to 10.

With each of these entries, try to describe the pain. What did it feel like? Was it aching, sharp, dull, throbbing, shooting, burning, electrical, or some sort of tingling sensation?

All of these subtle differences can help you make a self-diagnosis or help your doctor figure out the source of your pain a lot faster. Whenever a runner calls me for an online second opinion and I have all of this information, it really makes it a lot easier to help the runner get back on track faster.

When to make entries in your journal.

You need to track 3 basic times: 1) During the run. 2) The evening after the run and 3) the next morning after your run. This holds true for any activity. If you are just walking or doing an elliptical trainer, you want to keep track of what happens during the activity. How do you feel that evening following the activity, and how your foot first feels when you wake up and step out of bed next morning.

How long should runners track pain?

If you are running every day or even every other day, you can often see trends in as little as a few days, and almost certainly within two weeks. For that reason the Runner's Pain Journal we made for you is only 14 entries long. You can always print additional sheets if you need. But the reality is, you should be able to make progress quickly if you are paying close attention and making good choices as you heal.

Why runners should share pain with their doctor.

The more information you give your doctor, the easier it is for the doctor to make the correct diagnosis. The solution is often deep in the details. Part of the reason I have so much success with helping runners through online second opinions is that the runners have already been to one or two other doctors, and after those visits they seem to have started keeping better track of changes. They know better what has helped, and what hasn't. All of that information helps me rapidly hone in on the correct solution.

How to tell when it's okay to run.

Many doctors will say, "Just let pain be your guide." They imply that you have to expect to be pain free before you can. They suggest that you should be entirely pain free when you start running. But that isn't really the case.

The goal isn't to be pain free. The goal is to have less and less pain as you have more and more activity. You have to understand the difference between acceptable pain and worrisome pain.

If your pain has been decreasing to the point where it is almost gone, and you have no tenderness, its likely safe to start ramping up your activity.

How to tell when it's okay to increase distance and intensity.
The bottom line is you need to be able to increase your activity, build your strength, get stronger and run farther without having you pain ramp back up.

You have to consider your timing, your goals and then do everything you can to maintain your fitness.

Generally speaking, if you can run without swelling, without bruising coming back and without your pain returning or building again, then it is probably okay to run further and start adding in some intensity. But the specifics vary somewhat depending upon what specific structure is injured and your specific running goals.

That's why it's so important to find a doctor you can talk to who works with runners. Your doctor has to be on board with your goal of getting back to running. You and your doctor have to be on the same team.

Runner's Pain Journal as a prevention tool.

Almost never does an over-training injury happen in one instant. Most runners who call me for help will talk about the "sudden" injury, but then admit they felt a subtle dull ache or some minor nagging pain for days or weeks or even months that was gradually getting worse.

Keeping track of any pain or soreness will allow you to notice the trends in discomfort that can build over time. The earlier you identify the pain, the easier it is to prevent the true catastrophe that can keep you from running.

The more closely you track and evaluate your pain as you recover, the faster you can adjust, increase your mileage and ramp up your running intensity without having to wonder whether or not you are staying on track.

Again, the goal is to keep increasing your mileage and intensity without the pain creeping back in.

You can really only do that if you are keeping track with a pain journal.

To make things easy for you, I already created the perfect Runners Pain Journal PDF for you. It's on the next page. Just print out the next page and use it.

References: 1. Tesarz J, Schuster AK, Hartmann M, Gerhardt A, Eich W. Pain perception in athletes compared to normally active controls: A systematic review with meta-analysis PAIN, June 2012. Vol 153; #6, p. 1253-1262.

Runner's Pain Journal

Run Date	Run distance & location (trail, treadmill, concrete, asphalt)	Rate Run Intensity scale of 1-10	Where was the pain? (top of foot, heel, arch, Achilles, ankle, shin, ball of foot)	How much pain during run scale of 1-10	Did it get better, worse or stay same throughout the run?	Did pain go away during run? If so, at what mile?	Did pain come back later? If so, at what mile?	How much pain in evening after run?	How much pain in morning after run?	Describe (aching, sharp, dull, throbbing, shooting, burning, electrical, tingling)

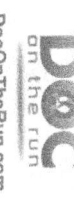

DocOnTheRun.com

Appendix 2
Recovering Runner's Next Step

THE NEXT STEP: GET INJURY SPECIFIC HELP...

Every little thing you do to increase your rate of healing, or decrease the tissue damage that can potentially setback your recovery...it all matters.

Over the last 15 years of working specifically with injured runners I have lectured to thousands of physicians at medical conferences to help them understand how to treat injured runners better. I have also helped countless professional, elite and recreational runners like you heal faster and get back on the fast track to recovery.

During all that time I've created hundreds of video lessons, podcast episodes and other self-help resources just to help you understand all the tips and tricks I use with elite athletes to get them back to running faster.

The fastest way for you to access all of those resources is to take the 30-Second Injured Runner Quiz to help you understand your injury better. Get immediate help access here: **https://www.docontherun.com/quiz**

FINAL THOUGHT

THIS MOMENT IS THE BEGINNING OF A NEW DAY.
WHEN TOMORROW COMES,
TODAY WILL BE GONE FOREVER,
LEAVING IN ITS PLACE SOMETHING YOU HAVE TRADED FOR IT.

WHAT YOU DO TODAY MATTERS.
TODAY YOU CAN GET WEAKER, OR STRONGER.
TODAYS' CHOICES WILL HELP YOUR BODY HEAL FASTER OR SLOWER.
THE DECISIONS YOU MAKE ALL DAY MAY EACH SEEM INSIGNIFICANT,
BUT WILL ALL ADD UP TO EITHER SUCCESS OR FAILURE.
IT'S YOUR CHOICE. RECOVER WISELY.

THE MOST INCREDIBLE FREE GIFT EVER ...ONLY FOR RECOVERING RUNNERS.

CONGRATULATIONS ON MAKING IT ALL THE WAY THROUGH THROUGH THE RUNNING INJURY ROADMAP!

I realize that your most valuable resource is time and you dedicated valuable time to reading something I wrote for you, so you could better understand exactly where you are along you're running injury recovery journey. I hope I haven't squandered that opportunity. I am grateful for your attention.

SINCE YOU MADE IT THIS FAR I WANT TO GIVE YOU A TRULY VALUABLE FREE GIFT.

I WOULD LIKE TO OFFER YOU THE OPPORTUNITY TO TAKE ALL OF WHAT YOU LEARNED AND TAKE IT ONE STEP FURTHER.

THIS IS 7-DAY ACCESS TO A 100% FREE TRIAL OF THE DOC ON THE RUN TRAINING SITE.

HERE YOU WILL BE ABLE TO ACCESS FREE TRAININGS, RESOURCES AND GUIDES YOU JUST CAN'T GET ANYWHERE ELSE.

($3,576 OF RUNNING SPECIFIC HELP)

YOU WILL GET IMMEDIATE ACCESS SELF-HELP COURSES, CHALLENGES AND RESOURCES THAT WILL HELP YOU RETURN TO RUNNING FASTER.

I am not asking you to say "yes."

Just say "maybe" and get it all for free right now.

Go to

www.DocOnTheRun.com/freegift

www.ingramcontent.com/pod-product-compliance
Lightning Source LLC
Chambersburg PA
CBHW050442010526
44118CB00013B/1648